MOTHER NATURE'S A BITCH

A guide to prolonging a quality life

Steven J. Block M.D.

ISBN: 0692445846
ISBN 13: 9780692445846
Library of Congress Control Number: 2015912337
Steven J. Block M.D., Stockton, CA

To the three most important people in my life . . .
Melanie, Jenna and Vanessa

TABLE OF CONTENTS

DISCLAIMER:
HONESTY IS THE BEST POLICY

This is not a scientific work. There are no footnotes and relatively few references to scientific studies. The reason? Surely it's not to fool the reader into accepting my speculations and conclusions as absolute. From my viewpoint, biological science is not exact because our knowledge is ever expanding and, knowing only part of the story, one can't guarantee the ending. So, what we believe with self-deceiving assuredness today, may be only partially correct or even downright wrong tomorrow. And, then there is that endless production of medical literature, which I dare say is often meticulously generated and completely worthless to the average human being trying to live a healthier and longer life. So that while the induction of a rapid and irregular heart rhythm in a fly may be fascinating to the funded team from the University of the Absurd, the average "Joe" or "Jill" really doesn't give a crap.

Before my first day at medical school in 1967, I borrowed several medical journals from the library. I guess my inflated ego, or perhaps my insecurities, somehow directed my decision to read a few dissertations on random medical subjects, one or more of which, my naiveté speculated, might just be the holy grail of medical school success. That evening, I had a great deal of trouble selecting which article might be more important than another; every one seemed critical, so I read all of them. Compulsively, I felt obligated to study and memorize every significant point as if there was a lesson in each that I might someday call upon to save the life of a future patient.

Exhausted from a night of serious reading, and fulfilling a routine obligation, I and a small group of fellow students met with the Chief of the Surgical Service. The purpose of the encounter was purely introductory and not academic. At the conclusion of the welcoming shtick, I noticed a tall stack of journals on the Chief's desk. Enough articles to occupy me through at least the first full year of medical school. When he asked if there were any questions, I couldn't resist and asked, "How do you read all that medical literature and have time for anything else?" His response was a demonstration of expert hand-eye coordination and verbal agility. He fingered through the contents of nearly a dozen journals with lightening speed, providing commentary attesting to the practical importance of certain articles, the silliness of others and even what he perceived as an author's poor track record for honesty, including denials of conflict of interest. My take home message from the meeting was that experience is paramount when you're dealing with an overabundance of data and opinion in a world where distinction is often defined by *how much* you publish, or earn, rather than *what* you publish, or how honestly you earned it.

So, here I am after nearly four decades of private medical practice, unwilling to give it up without sharing my perspective on what's important and what's not in a medical society drowning in its literature, and a lay public bombarded by "scientific" claims that, if taken as absolute truth, often accomplish nothing except the transfer of hard-earned money into the pockets of pilferers.

I have selected topics that are routinely raised by my patients with remarkable consistency. My calling is louder than ever as I accept my label as "senior" and more clearly recognize that Mother Nature is a bitch! But she deserves that label only from the viewpoint of an audacious species that wants to live forever, feeling and acting like they deserve perpetual health and physical prime.

INTRODUCTION

Natural Selection is a term that will appear in any work that explores evolution; whether the author believes that the process of mutation (which produces either beneficial or detrimental traits, the former favoring survival and the latter discouraging it) is entirely random or divinely inspired. For me, it makes no sense to embrace an uncompromising view of the mechanism that drives natural selection when logic is limited and the reality is equally consistent with chance, or a monotheistic force at the helm. Even Einstein denied he was an atheist, and wrote that while some might suggest he was an agnostic, he preferred "an attitude of humility corresponding to the weakness of our intellectual understanding of nature and our own being."

Why is Mother Nature a bitch? She's not vulgar or vile, but rather doing her job as best she can. Her task (or assignment from an all-powerful source) is to retain each species at any cost. This survival of the fittest makes good sense even if it is often cruel. Some of the excess young with minor defects, or the old (realistically defined as any organism no longer capable of reproduction) need to die in order to prevent less-than-ideal traits from entering the gene pool, and help preserve the food supply for the sexually active. At first glance, one might easily assume that for Mother Nature, using medication to treat *erectile dysfunction* in the male of a species, makes about as much sense as digging up a corpse for the sake of doing so. More on this subject later.

The purpose of this book is ***not*** to discourage the reader from basking in the light of medical discovery; on the contrary, human ingenuity, as we will explore, offers an opportunity to fool Mother Nature in a non-confrontational manner. She sat powerless as our species' brain capacity expanded, the reality offering those in her kingdom both a blessing and a curse. For every less than genetically perfect infant (defined as an individual lacking some trait that encouraged survival in the wild), there was the possibility of a nascent mind eventually capable of taming the elements and keeping predators, both gigantic and microscopic, in abeyance. She watches our every move and knows she has a powerful ally hidden in every cell of the human body–our DNA, whose essence remains more vintage than modern, maladjusted to the artificial extension of human life from its intended four or five decades. Her agenda then, comes into direct conflict with ours, and thus we watch our vitality wane with time and, fairly or not, label her unflatteringly. So, in the pages that follow, I will explore the human dilemma of the desire to live indefinitely in Mother Nature's world, which touts our programmed reality that says, "not so fast," and in the process, offer my suggestions (tricks if you like) that might just add quality years to your life.

WHY DO I AGE?

Getting old–a big part of her plan

O ur perception of the aging process transforms from nonexistence in childhood, to "the other guy's problem" in young adulthood, to "poor grandma and grandpa" in our thirties and forties, to a quiet, tentative self-deception of invulnerability as we approach and pass Social Security age, and finally to (with the help of a mirror) "crap, I'm running out of time." You know you're at least sort of old when the fantasies of writing that best-selling novel, entering politics to change the world, having that home that resembles the Hearst Castle, leave you. You know you're really old when there seems little difference amongst the choices of a burial plot in the ground, a final resting place above the ground, or cremation.

All this is quite irrelevant to Mother Nature, who remembers our species in the context of the 1600s when reaching age fifty was exceptional. She's accepting of modern reality and the dumb-luck mutations in our DNA that permitted the discovery of antibiotics, the methodology for sewage disposal, and the technology needed to exterminate large numbers of disease-carrying rodents.

She may even grin just a bit with a tough-love recognition that no near-sighted wildebeest, or arthritic zebra, or diabetic hyena, or morbidly obese giraffe ever survived long enough to pollute her gene pool. But, there is another reason for what some might call a suspicious smirk on her metaphoric face–***telomeres***!

Reducing the science of genetics to its simplest form, each individual human (except for identical twins) is unique based on his or her DNA–that material in the nucleus of every living cell in our bodies that directs all life processes from conception to death. Cells divide, replicating the identical coded message in each daughter cell that dictates its function. The code is also contained in egg and sperm cells, allowing the mixture of two distinct DNA complements to mingle in the production of offspring, which minimizes the duplication of partially expressed negative traits, avoiding a double dose of unhelpful characteristics, which is an obvious benefit for survival.

So, why do we notice Mother Nature's slightly sly countenance? She's booby-trapped our DNA by placing telomeres on the ends of each of our chromosomes. Often compared to aglets, or the plastic tips on the ends of shoelaces, telomeres protect the ends of DNA from deteriorating and eventually combining in ways that would be suicidal for the organism. But, ***with each cell division, telomeres shorten, and the reservoir of youth takes a hit as cellular stability declines***. One might be tempted to ask Mother Nature, "Why sanction this apparatus in the first place?" Her response might be twofold.

First, she would remind us that without telomeres, the existence of any meaningfully biologically stable organism would be impossible. Life would be exquisitely short and physically and metabolically chaotic, reproduction probably impossible.

Second, she might throw us a crumb and explain that something called ***telomerase*** exists by her grace. This enzyme repairs telomeres and prevents their shortening. I might briefly thank her, but also remind her that by prolonging cell life, there is a greater chance of mutation with an increased risk of cancer. Specifically, a recent analysis of individuals with a genetic variant associated with long telomeres demonstrated an increased risk for developing **glioma**, a type of brain tumor. Willing to answer us or not, by now **MN** (I'll call Mother Nature that from now on) is most likely annoyed: "Your mutated brain may be your curse. Your ego and arrogance, unique in the natural world, has transcended survival advantage. Figure it out for yourself!"

Now what? What practical advice can we take away from the telomere/telomerase reality, as we understand it today?

Simply use common sense and appreciate the concept of moderation. Be cautious. Unproven claims abound. Small pilot studies (watch out for the over-used, dirty little hooks, "clinically proven," or "our scientists have shown") are often deliberately misleading. Suggesting that the results of a small self-serving study represent established fact is <u>not</u> much different than claiming that when a baseball player with a zero batting average for the season finally gets a hit, the color of the batter's underwear, or the catcher's new credit card number (or any other condition at the time) was directly responsible for the ballplayer's success. This questionable reasoning appears daily in our lives on television, radio, in newspaper and magazine ads. We are inundated with health claims that have no basis in proven fact and conveniently hide behind the tiny print requiring a microscope to read, which advises, "***<u>This statement has not been evaluated by the Food and Drug Administration. This product is not intended to diagnose, treat or cure, or prevent any disease</u>***." Or, as greater honesty would dictate: "God bless the placebo effect and the fortunes it creates," or perhaps just, "There's a sucker born every minute."

You'll hear or read claims that suggest telomeres are particularly vulnerable to the process of oxidation and inflammation–perhaps. But, to suggest that a wide variety of antioxidants (vitamins, minerals, plant phenols, etc.) lengthen telomeres or delay their shortening is pure speculation and a gimmick to sell products. These unproven assertions are not unlike saying we can stop acid rain by gargling with baking soda.

It is clear that the telomere/telomerase interaction with human longevity and disease is substantially more complex than currently understood. Those selling products prefer not to recognize that deficiency. But, there has been recent work out of UCSF that suggests simple *lifestyle changes* can result in measurable increases in telomere length.

A diet low in processed foods and fat and rich in plant foods, as well as moderate physical exercise, stress reduction, and more social support and affection, resulted in a 10% increase in telomere length, while the control group demonstrated a slight shortening over the same period of time.

Now, let's look at this objectively. The mechanism responsible for this lengthening remains unclear. And having more sex is quite different than choosing a wholegrain cereal. But, all the lifestyle changes discussed make common sense and are proposed in moderation (*the study required 20 to 30 minutes of walking for their "moderate" exercise*). If you examine our dentition, appreciate the incredibly complex interaction of our bones, joints and tendons, recognize the stress in our intricate lives and appreciate how critical a stable family and social environment was to the survival of our distant ancestors, it seems a no-brainer that the recommended lifestyle changes certainly, in the words of my grandmother, "couldn't hurt."

IS TESTOSTERONE THERAPY SAFE?

Testosterone con hits below and above the belt

L et's not kid ourselves; the testosterone molecule is probably second only to highly enriched uranium in its contribution to the potential destruction of our, and all, species inhabiting the planet. MN might raise a metaphoric eyebrow with fleeting doubt. After all, without this male hormone there would, at the very least, be no male maturation and no production of sperm, or, with admitted speculation, a species resembling us might have evolved, reproducing offspring by budding like *hydra* (a tiny fresh-water animal). But I suspect that MN would soon nod in agreement. Male leaders hold the grand prize for screwing up human history from its earliest recording. Even before that, our prehistoric ancestors' *Y chromosomes* gave them bigger muscles that urged them to confront any stranger (particularly male) from outside the immediate clan. This "assignment" as physically stronger hunter, as opposed to less physically strong gatherer (male versus female), is not only responsible for nascent spousal abuse, but probably a subliminal desire to defeat the "enemy" at any cost. Not all that different from male elk aggressiveness during the rutting season.

But, this is not to selectively chastise a particular hormone in a series of molecules necessary for our very existence. It's merely an attempt to set the context for yet another example of how our brainpower has corrupted biological necessity.

In the male human, testosterone blood levels vary with age. Measuring these levels in ng/dL units, minimal amounts are detected until approximately age 12. At age 14, the levels are usually still low, but by ages 15 to 16, they start to rise. On average, these levels tend to peak between ages 17 and 18. One might wonder why the hell MN is driving these psychologically vulnerable, fledging humans into non-stop sexual obsession. MN might respond simply: "If you're supposed to live to only forty or so, you better get busy making babies, or kiss your species good-bye."

The average adult human male between age 20 and 39, has a serum testosterone level that varies widely from about 270 to 1,070 units. From mid-thirties on, there is an expected 1% drop per year. For comparison, the normal range for serum sodium is 135 to 145 mEq/L, which is clearly much narrower. Few blood measurements in humans have such a wide range of what is considered "normal" as the testosterone level. So, men can have nearly four times more or less and are still considered "normal." For me, as a physician, it sends a message that *low testosterone levels* (or *low "T"*) should be diagnosed with great caution.

There are many reasons for depression, fatigue, and decreased libido in men over forty other than low "T." In my practice, I routinely send patients with these symptoms and low, or low normal, levels of testosterone to an *endocrinologist* for additional evaluation.

I am driven nearly insane with the never-ending television commercials for remedies for *erectile dysfunction* (*ED*). While listening to the news, all I need to hear is the preliminary music and I change the channel. These intrusions are so omnipresent that I even recognize the orchestra that the marketing people use when it's a commercial unrelated to ED. Added to this massive, and highly successful, campaign to link loving wives' little quirks with a primitive, and appropriate, response of jumping her bones for immediate sexual gratification, and the macho man who can steer a boat through a Category 5 hurricane, or the grease-covered guy who can single-handedly reconstruct a demolished Mac Truck with his bare hands and a screwdriver, comes the opportunistic bombardment of products that will raise your testosterone levels, cure your depression, moodiness and fatigue, and boost your sickly libido. So, it is in this context of a media blitz that male patients, somewhat reluctantly, and nearly always at the end of an office visit, meekly ask what I think about *Viagra, Levitra, Cialis*, and *testosterone gels*.

What if we asked MN what she thinks? She'd probably mock impotence therapies. After all, the species likes to fly even though its members have no wings. And besides, a user of this "therapy" might just drop dead from asymptomatic coronary disease – no loss there.

Regarding supplemental testosterone, MN would probably remind us that while most men over forty can procreate, they have no damn business doing so because they're not only lucky to be alive, but may carry significant mutations in their sperm. [It's no longer thought that just older women may carry genetic defects in their ova (eggs)]. Unlike other mutations in younger men, which may have helped dumb creatures turn into smart-asses, these biological aberrations in older men are more likely to add destructive elements to the gene pool. Furthermore, MN might explain that if a man messes with hormones that are intended to diminish with age, there are major biological consequences. I would agree, since there is solid scientific evidence suggesting that ___raising testosterone levels artificially is associated with enlarging your prostate, increasing the risk of prostate cancer, and increasing your risk for both heart attack and stroke___. This pessimistic message, by FDA demand, must accompany these commercials. But let's be real–the poor guy, who's hesitant to look his wife of thirty or forty years of marriage in the eye for fear that she might hint at an interest in intimacy (because he'd have to consult his diary for the last time he experienced an erection), has little concern for the amicably spoken risks of the product when he watches the magic bottle of product rise like a teenager's woodie in a panorama of masculine machines moving overhead, promising the male species can do anything; and, all the while, MN giggles.

But, in all fairness to an important, normal human desire (not to mention the purpose of this book), there is a monumental difference between testosterone supplementation and the use of FDA-approved medications for erectile dysfunction.

Blood vessels constrict or dilate as an adaptive mechanism, providing greater circulation to biologically more active regions of our bodies. Think about it. You're sitting at a table at a wedding reception after a five-course dinner that contained enough calories to sustain a wildebeest on its annual migration. Your stomach is so full that even the thought of a sip of water seems like torture. In this setting, MN has maximized the blood flow to your gastrointestinal tract to facilitate digestion, appropriately "sacrificing" circulation to your leg muscles, which don't need much in their state of suspended animation. (Pray that the bride doesn't ask you to the dance floor to explore her latest Zumba dance moves).

This biologically sound redistribution of blood, by need, is accomplished through a number of mechanisms, one of which involves a substance called, ***cyclic guanosine monophosphate***, or ***cGMP***. This compound relaxes smooth muscle in arterial walls, dilating the vessels and increasing circulation.

As in all complex biological systems, one effect counters another; the balance established is a stabilizing force crucial for survival in any living organism. In this case, cGMP (the stuff that increases circulation) is metabolized (broken down to an <u>ineffective</u> product before elimination from the body) by a number of substances called *phosphodiesterases (or PDEs). Viagra (sildenafil), Levitra (ava-nafil) and Cialis (tadalafil)* are *inhibitors* of one of these "break-down" substances (specifically *PDE 5*).

Simply put, you ingest any of these agents to treat ED and they interfere with one of the mechanisms that <u>counter</u> the effects that increase circulation. The result is more circulation to the organ where you want it. These ED drugs are not entirely targeted to the penis. The above-mentioned medications have effects elsewhere in the human body, and thus can dilate blood vessels in other organs and, in some cases of patients with abnormally constricted blood vessels in the lungs (called *pulmonary hypertension*), may lower the pressure and improve symptoms. Furthermore, since vasodilata-tion (opening an artery, allowing more blood flow) is accomplished by more than a single pathway, other medications that can lower blood pressure (most importantly <u>*nitrates*</u> and blood-pressure low-ering agents called *alpha blockers*, or *alpha antagonists,* (see sec-tion: "IS LOWER BLOOD PRESSURE ALWAYS BETTER? *Going beyond therapeutic?*") can have additive effects that can drop blood pressure to dangerously low levels.

So, what's the take home message here? *While I believe that testosterone itself should only be taken after a thorough work-up by a qualified physician with a background in endocrinology, and after the substantial risks are explored in detail, medications for ED (with the precautions I've outlined) have a legitimate role to play in modern medicine.* You see, there's a difference between a metaphoric MN's disdain for the "process" or motivation for the use of medications for ED and the biological effect on a male genome (all his chro-mosomes or inherited traits). Look, *if we're trying to "trick" MN into thinking we're still able to reproduce prime offspring, a "zero" sex life is not the answer. It's logical that our DNA is more likely to turn on favorable genes and turn off unfavorable genes if the essential act in the procreation of any species is alive, and (if not exactly "well") at least functional.*

VITAMINS . . . TOO MUCH OF A GOOD THING?

Voodoo vitamins and other deceptions

If MN possessed even a hint of empathy, or sympathy, for humankind (and was willing to corrupt her respect for cattle, her bovine creations that have no propensity to abuse her), she might have a cow over this subject.

Let's begin with a clear understanding of what the hell *vitamins* really are! They are a hodgepodge of unrelated organic compounds (substances that contain nitrogen) that are needed by the body in *tiny* amounts, and act as *coenzymes* or *cofactors* (molecules that hook up with proteins to assist or permit their function), or assume a form that must be biochemically acted upon to become a coenzyme. The key word here is "tiny," as in minute or miniscule. These substances are generally available in adequate quantities in foods consumed in normal amounts.

I can see our metaphoric MN nodding approval and then getting angry. I can almost hear her object: "You are the product of millions of years of genetic mutation and evolution. Your DNA is my masterpiece where every stroke has been painted in perfect harmony with survival. And what do you do with your superior brains? You finger paint over my canvas."

Let's explore her objections: vitamins are divided into **water-soluble** (vitamins C and B Complex), or **fat-soluble** (vitamins A, D, E and K). Your kidneys readily dump the former (our European friends often joke about how expensive our urine is); the latter (fat soluble) are absorbed more slowly, require **bile** as a detergent for absorption, and are stored in the body.

In regard to **vitamin C**, it is true that if our species decides to explore the oceans by ancient ship, extending our relatively feeble prowess in the water to transcontinental investigation, and the galley doesn't provide vitamin-C-containing fruits and vegetables on the long voyage, the absence of this **cofactor** (vitamin C), which is responsible for a number of reactions that make **collagen** (the fibrous protein that holds various body tissues together), will cause muscles to ache, skin to bruise, teeth to loosen, and eventually convulsions and death.

How much vitamin C do we need? It appears that about **50 mg per day prevents scurvy. I estimate that 100 mgs per day, or twice that amount, is a good idea.** Now comes the controversy. What's the best, **highest dose** one should take for maximal health benefit without adverse consequences?

To begin with, absorption studies provide a hint: The more vitamin C you take orally, the less you absorb. It's as if MN, in a moment of weakness, has provided us with both a mechanism we're less likely to screw up and a warning against excess.

Vitamin C is touted as an **anti-oxidant** (a term often heard on the airwaves, or spelled out in magazines, or on food packages with the intent of corrupting our psyche into equating the designation with youth, health, agelessness, and maybe a better chance at winning the lottery). **What this (anti-oxidation) means is that when fat is broken down to provide energy, it creates a chemical circumstance where**

an "unshared" electron exists. This chemically hungry guy (called a *free radical* – no relationship to amnesty for political prisoners) readily reacts with oxygen and forms a damage-causing product called a **Reactive Oxygen Species** or **ROS**. This is a" bad" thing, counterbalanced by a variety of "good" reactions, which are built into the complicated interactions that take place in a living organism, the specifics of which are of great interest to those few of us whose love of life is synonymous with bright fluorescent lights, soundproof cubbies and grant money. So, why not load up with vitamin C and stop those ROSs? The reason is that *vitamin C has the potential to act as a pro-oxidant, at least in a test tube.*

While controversial, the chemical possibility that vitamin C might act as a pro-oxidant raises the concern that too-high doses of it might backfire, causing the formation of superoxide-like reactive oxygen species, which can really mess up one's plans to outlive their pet parrot. More specifically, there have been small studies, which have suggested high doses of vitamin C may accelerate hardening of the carotid arteries in the necks of the elderly, and perhaps even damage DNA in certain blood cells.

So, what should we do? Recognizing the function of vitamins in general, understanding that in the case of vitamin C, absorption is inversely proportional to the amount consumed, respecting that our current medical knowledge is still primitive relative to what is still unknown, I generally advise my patients *not to exceed 2000 mgs of vitamin C per day in supplements.* If only MN was a patient and I could look into her eyes for a clue as to the ideal dose.

Vitamin E is a fat-soluble vitamin, which means there must be some level of fat in your small bowel in order for absorption to take place; this is usually no problem even if one is following a low-fat diet.

There are multiple chemical variations of vitamin E, but for the purpose of this discussion I will focus exclusively on the form called **alpha-tocopherol**. This is not only the usual molecular structure present in supplements, but is preferentially selected (over other ingested forms) by the liver for entry into our blood stream. It also has been the protagonist employed in nearly all clinical studies assessing its potential value (or detriment) in a number of disease entities.

First of all, let's look at properties it possesses [at least in the test tube (called *in vitro*)] that made it a tempting candidate for study. It's an **anti-oxidant** (there's that word again that nearly brings tears of joy to our eyes), which means, as in the case of vitamin C, it has the biological potential "power" to reduce those nasty **ROSs** that we don't want hanging around and doing their damage.

Since vitamin E is fat soluble, its potential benefit would seem even greater than the water-soluble vitamin C's, since fat-solubility means vitamin E is more likely to do things in, or on, **cellular membranes** (the chemically active biological envelope surrounding cells). This potentially helpful membrane activity probably applies to all cells and so, it's not surprising that researchers were motivated to test the long-term effects of vitamin E on the incidence of cancer and Alzheimer's disease, for example. Furthermore, since vitamin E seems to have an effect on gene expression (one of which may augment the "clean-up" of cholesterol that abnormally accumulates in hardening of the arteries), it was logical to look into the effects of this vitamin on vascular disease. The motivation to do so is further encouraged by vitamin E's apparent effect of discouraging the "sticking" of certain blood elements (called **platelets**), which can trigger blood clotting and precipitate heart attacks or strokes.

Okay, one important study to test the potential value of vitamin E (400 IU selected as the daily dose) in preventing coronary artery disease was called the **Heart Outcomes Prevention Evaluation Study** (or **HOPE**). It recruited nearly 10,000 patients (men and women), age 55 or older, all of whom were considered at high risk for coronary artery disease based on previously diagnosed vascular disease, or diabetes, and one additional risk factor (for example, high blood pressure or cigarette smoking). While the study was also interested in testing whether a medication for high blood pressure (an ACE inhibitor–more later in another section) was helpful, the design allowed for the legitimate testing of the effects of vitamin E on the incidence of heart attack, stroke, death by any cardiac event, unstable chest pain (from coronary artery disease called *angina pectoris*), coronary artery bypass surgery (or *angioplasty*–the opening of a blocked vessel with a balloon, usually followed by the insertion of a *stent* to keep it open), heart failure, amputation, death for any reason, complications of diabetes and cancer.

The *HOPE* study lasted an average of 4 ½ years. The results? Vitamin E did *no more* or *no less* than "sugar" pills! So, now what? Well, the HOPE study researchers got about 4,000 of the original cast members to continue the protocol (despite the unimpressive results) for another 2 ½ years, renaming the study *HOPE–TOO* (I doubt the promise of free vitamin E for life swayed many into participating). And guess what? After the extra time on vitamin E (now around 7 years total), the results were equally unimpressive, except for one unexpected outcome. Those extra two years of vitamin E, in this group of high-risk patients, was associated with a significant *increase* in hospitalization for *heart failure*! Go figure.

Another study enrolled 40,000 healthy women (no evidence of vascular disease), age 45 or older. They received 600 IU of vitamin E every other day or a placebo. The study continued for approximately a decade. When the researchers looked at a combined analysis (that is, *lumped together* all the bad outcomes they were investigating–non-fatal heart attacks, strokes and deaths from heart disease), once again vitamin E (in this "healthy" female population) was no more effective in doing good stuff as sugar pills. But, when they delved more deeply into the results, they did find that in these previously healthy women at the time of their entry into the study, there *was* a benefit. Now focus on this to avoid confusion. When they "pulled out" deaths from heart disease and non-fatal heart attacks, each *separately*, there was a benefit, particularly in those women age 65 or older. The authors entertained a number of suggestions for this positive finding, but a clear, final conclusion was never offered. Statistical analysis can be misleading, especially when the methods used are complex. *But it's my guess that the older participants, at higher risk for vascular disease than the younger participants, may have benefited from the anti-blood-clotting effects of vitamin E.*

One final study involving physicians (yes, sometimes "do as I say, not as I do" breaks down). In this one, 15,000 doctors, considering themselves healthy, age 50 or older, took *400 IU of vitamin E* (with 500 mgs of vitamin C), or placebo, for an average of 8 years. The results? Almost *nada*. *Vitamin E* and placebo's performance were consistent relative to the incidence of adverse cardiac outcomes, but the group taking the vitamin had a significantly higher likelihood of developing a stroke involving a bleed into the brain. This may be related to anti-platelet effects attributed to *vitamin E* as alluded to earlier in this section. *So maybe this effect helped older women, but was a detriment to middle-aged doctors?*

Cancer studies involving *vitamin E* supplementation have generally been negative, often confusing and occasionally mixed. One concern gleaned from a ton of data suggests that men taking 400 IU of vitamin E chronically may increase their risk for prostate cancer.

Eye studies attempting to ascertain any positive effects of *vitamin E* supplementation on the onset or progression of *cataracts* or *macular degeneration* have also been mixed.

Finally, and with no surprise, the anti-oxidant effects of *vitamin E* beg for an evaluation regarding its possible benefits in delaying the onset or the progression of *dementia* or *Alzheimer's disease*. Again, the studies (in my opinion nearly impossible to control properly when symptoms act like moving targets) have been mixed at best.

My personal opinion (based on current research and my understanding of the proposed mechanisms–not to mention my intuition regarding MN's "motives") is that it is **highly unlikely vitamin E** can have a significantly positive effect on these devastating central nervous system diseases when the very basis for our "unnatural" survival resides in that most complex of organs (our brain), uniquely subjecting itself to malfunction. To propose that a single vitamin with anti-oxidant properties can avert or delay this deterioration is like suggesting that a drop of oil in the right place can prevent a nuclear facility from meltdown.

Okay, to the practical. First of all, a diet high in **vitamin E** is a good idea. This can be accomplished with a greater emphasis on consuming items like **sunflower seeds or sunflower oil, almonds or peanuts. Vegetables high in Vitamin E include spinach and broccoli.** If you must take a supplement, I would recommend, for an adult, **no more than 100 IU a day**, unless there are extenuating circumstances worth a discussion with your doctor. Note, this 100 IU dose is more than four times the minimal daily requirement.

I've only covered two of the most popular supplements in detail with the hope that you will appreciate the hidden intricacies the marketers of such products don't want you to know. Vitamins play a critical role in sustaining a healthy life, but remember **there's a difference between quenching your thirst and drowning.** As I mentioned earlier, commercials for these products protect themselves with the often-microscopic disclaimer that the FDA hasn't evaluated their claims. This cop out means nothing less than these companies can say whatever they damn well please and their asses are protected. Remember, these for-profit enterprises usually lasso a speck of truth, or a perceived public conception (not infrequently, public misconception), and milk it dry with expert marketing. **_There's a difference between truth and relevancy, and an even bigger difference between isolated truth and relevancy_**.

A variation on this theme of faux sciences is the manipulation of numbers. Ever notice that advertisers never ascribe a percentage benefit attributed to their product in numbers ending in zero? This vitamin-enriched crème reduces ugly brown spots on your skin by 57%. Or this unique combination of minerals (and secret sauce) improves memory by an amazing 83%. They do this because numbers ending in zero seem so unscientific, so arbitrary, so bourgeois. Now throw in an odd number and the potential purchaser will be convinced that this so-called "clinical" study is the real thing, even though the participants were all employees of the company selling the product and self-reported the incredible benefits. A legitimate clinical study recruits large numbers of patients carefully screened to avoid individual characteristics that might complicate the end points (clinical outcomes) and, if feasible, double-blinds the investigation, which means neither researcher nor patient participant knows who got the sugar pill and who got the real deal.

One final note on what both politicians and the general public too often downgrade to "benign" treachery. When a particular vitamin is associated with a certain legitimate benefit (the benefit often not realistically applicable to anyone, except someone near starvation), the ad people seize the opportunity to push new products, which are usually not new at all, but rather just another slight variation in the game they play. So, for example, let's say that the public perceives, correctly so, that vitamin A is good for one's eyes. Well, despite the fact that there are already a ton of products with more than adequate amounts of the supplement in a variety of available formulations, this presents a potential marketing opportunity. Pick a preferably inexpensive mineral, or cheap root available in the back lot, throw it into the vitamin A mix, package it with class, and generate a new ad campaign that praises MN for the gift of sight, providing the viewer with images of our miraculous sense of vision. With thankful tears in those special organs we've so callously neglected, the good-intentioned patsy heads to the store and buys, at a premium, a designer eye supplement that probably differs minimally, (certainly biologically insignificantly), from what he or she is already taking, and carries it home, adding it to the fortune of products already in the medicine cabinet. This protected (not entirely dishonest) con, can best be seen by selling supplements to various age groups, suggesting that if we plan graduating to a higher level of survival, we must have the correct school supplies. This gets even worse when the products for sale contain substances that no one, not even a Chinese wizard, let alone the FDA, has the slightest idea of what the hell is in them, and even less of an idea about their effects. So, beware of a product specially formulated to dissolve blockages in your arteries, derived from a secret Incan remedy lost for centuries [until discovered by Dr. Stockoption, (and strongly recommended by MN)], with a money-back guarantee that it will keep you alive for 100 years, if you are not completely satisfied, or hospitalized, or dead, whichever comes last.

CAN ASPIRIN SAVE ME FROM A HEART ATTACK OR STROKE?

Aspirin–pissing off Mother Nature

In the incalculable, evolutionary complexities that made a human out of a single-celled living organism, let's focus on one. If you're going to walk upright, dig in soil for roots to eat, or carry a sharpened stick for hunting, there's a damn good chance something may go wrong: your foot catches on a vine or you slip in mud and you go down on your backside; your bare hand finds a sharp unseen stone and you cut your finger; your hungry best buddy's enthusiasm for the kill and dinner puts his spear through both his prey and your foot. Trouble in the "paradise" of early man? Not necessarily. That's because MN has provided our species with a mechanism to stop the bleeding before we exsanguinate. When our blood vessels (both miniscule and large) are traumatized, a ballet of biochemical reactions comes into play with the end result, the formation of a blood clot that stops the bleeding. (See section: "WHAT'S THAT FLUTTER IN MY CHEST? *Atrial fibrillation—a valentine from Mother Nature*").

The initial step in the process of normal ***coagulation*** (blood clotting) involves tiny fragments of circulating cells called ***platelets*** (we mentioned them when discussing vitamin E), which essentially stick to the damaged inner lining of the vessel and initiate a complex series of events.

Platelets originate in the bone marrow from large cells (called ***megakaryocytes***) where they, and other blood cell elements, mature from ***stem cells***. Their "adult" forms are released into the circulation. This is a pretty classy deal from which MN can take pride as she protects her young and fertile breeders from disabling or fatal hemorrhaging.

Then comes this guy from Oxford in 1763, who, from her standpoint, literally barks up the wrong tree (a willow tree to be exact) and discovers a chemical that, with some minor adjustment, the world will eventually know as ***aspirin***. So, why is she pissed? It would seem, at first, that MN's wrath might be more realistically placed had the guy discovered a double cheeseburger topped with fried onions and an attached coupon for a free angioplasty. But, with further thought, her reaction is more understandable. If humans' expanded brains lead them to bad choices and they die, that's a good thing in that it removes them from the gene pool before they pollute it any further. Aspirin has an ***anti-platelet*** effect that discourages blood clot formation, particularly in smaller vessels. The process of ***atherosclerosis***, or hardening of the arteries, can begin very early in life. Its progression to clinical significance is highly variable and affected significantly by genetics and accelerated by uncontrolled high blood pressure, smoking, diabetes, obesity, inactivity and, perhaps most importantly, the level of ***LDL***, or so-called "bad" cholesterol. (See section: "CAN DRUGS KEEP MY ARTERIES OPEN? ***Mother Nature's nemesis–the statin drugs***").

So, what's the story with MN's indignation? ***Aspirin***, by inhibiting platelets from sticking to the roughened surfaces of partially blocked blood vessels infiltrated by bad cholesterol and the detrimental cellular consequences thereof, can prevent a blood clot from forming, and thus save an organ from damage (for example: prevent a heart attack if it's a coronary artery; prevent a stroke if it's a vessel in the brain; save bowel if it's a vessel supplying the small or large intestine). What she might say if confronted for an explanation is: "No creature in my kingdom in the wild ever dies from hardening of the arteries. Your brain has saved you from many of the perils I have placed in the arena of your existence for good reason. But the lifestyle you have created in defiance of my laws has paid you back with ailments that lessen the impact of your arrogance. And now, in further rebellion, you find a trick that robs me of the satisfaction of watching you pay for your biological sins."

Before my recommendation, it's important that you understand that in the complicated process of aspirin biochemistry, there is the inhibition of a protein (an enzyme) that plays an important role in protecting the lining of the stomach and small intestine. ***Thus, aspirin does increase the risk of bleeding (is that a wry smile I see on MN's face?) and is <u>not</u> for primary prevention of vascular disease in the general population. But, if you have no allergy to aspirin, no history of gastrointestinal intolerance or bleeding with its use, are not taking other blood thinners, and have a significant overall risk of vascular disease (as determined by your physician), I recommend 81 mgs (so-called low-dose or "baby") enteric coated aspirin daily.***

IS THERE AN EXERCISE THAT CAN SLOW THE CLOCK?

The muscle group that deceives Mother Nature

Survival requires a defensive strategy against predation. All living species have achieved an evolutionary state that permits enough individuals to reach maturity and generate offspring. The means by which this is accomplished is highly variable. One species may release so many fertilized eggs into the ocean that even if 99% are eaten, or don't hatch, there are still enough survivors to reach reproductive adulthood. Other species may have only one or just a few offspring, and protect them with extreme maternal or paternal ferocity.

Recently, after observing circling hawks at an unusually low altitude, I was overcome by a humanitarian obligation to rescue several feral kittens from a neighbor's woodpile. As I approached the section of logs, where I had seen one of the kittens disappear, the mother cat suddenly appeared blocking my forward progress. Obviously nursing, this five-pound feline glared at me with such fierceness that I stopped in my tracks. I regained my composure

and inched forward, confronted by an even more aggressive posture as if mother cat was going to leap for my jugular. I honesty felt
that the potential threat to her kittens had biochemically turned
on some latent gene that once graced the DNA of a saber-toothed
tiger. I postponed the rescue until later, waiting for mamma to go
on the hunt for something the size of a moose.

The point is that MN has instilled in every creature's genetic code the means to preserve its species. This is a dynamic process that does not exist in the vacuum of any particular biological
niche. Thousands, or even millions, of years of success guarantee
nothing. A neighbor's mutation can turn a benign nearby resident
into a life-threatening enemy overnight in evolutionary terms. But,
during periods of stability within a given species, the "survival"
gene or genes within the nuclei of each cell in the creature's body
empowers the organism with the means for a potentially winnable
fight, or a usually effective flight. When MN recognizes increasing
age, as **telomeres** shrink, she "expects" these mechanisms to fail.
The individual with arthritic joints, scarred lungs and hardened
coronary arteries is not only a sad biological enigma, but (if still
able to reproduce) also a dramatically unattractive donor of eggs
or sperm. In essence, MN must think: "Please die already. Save
the food for the young." So how does all this apply to "the muscle
group that deceives?"

The answer, the epiphany, came to me after I reflected on my
high school track experience. I was a 440-yard (now 400 meter)
runner. I was pretty good at it, but not great. And this reality probably contributed to my insecurity. Every race I ran in competition
followed a similar pattern: nervous as hell with no appetite twenty-
four hours before the event; warming up in front of the crowd of
onlookers, suppressing the urge to vomit (the chess team seeming
a better option as an extra-curricular); standing at the starting
line praying, not to win, but hoping not to fall or die; hearing
the gun and starting at ill-advised maximal speed; negotiating the

first turn and foolishly thinking this was a piece of cake after all; running down the backstretch, wondering how I could have so completely deceived myself; turning for home and the finish line, my body suddenly as independent of my mind as if my torso and arms belonged to a rag doll; and finally, experiencing excruciating pain in my **hamstring muscles (*semitendinosus, semimembranosus and biceps femoris*)**, crossing the finish line, panting as if a preview to a death rattle, more from the agony in my legs than an oxygen deficit, or metabolic acidosis.

It was my recollection of those high school athletic events that provided the clue. Think about it. Our species is not covered in poisonous spines, nor do we have scent glands like a skunk, nor the capability of changing color like a chameleon. If our DNA is programmed for a life span of not much more than four or five decades, and our primary mechanism to avoid predation is to run like hell, and when we do run like hell we preferentially work our hamstring muscles into severe pain, that must send a biochemical signal that we are still capable of fleeing and, by biological association, are probably youthful enough to warrant a go at reproducing without introducing some nasty, decayed gene.

So, here's the bottom line. I recommend that everyone **routinely exercise his or her hamstring muscles.** This can be accomplished with or without weights and machines. Strengthening these muscles just might deceive MN into believing you're younger than what your birth certificate indicates.

A recent article was published in a highly respected journal that followed more than 55,000 patients from 1974 through 2003. Entry required no history of baseline heart attack, stroke or cancer. All participants were questioned regarding their physical activities, specifically their running habits. Guess what? **Participants who ran just over ten minutes a day substantially reduced their risk of all-cause and cardiac mortality.** The benefits were clear, irrespective of age, sex, body habitus, general health, smoking history and alcohol use.

Not running contributed to mortality nearly as significantly as high blood pressure. It seems both biologically reasonable, and logical, that ***not walking*** (when one is capable of the activity) would likely impose a similar, negative outcome.

HOW CAN I KEEP
MY BRAIN YOUNG?

Dementia/Alzheimer's–Mother Nature's revenge

So, MN says to us, (beating around the bush, not her thing), "Okay smartasses, keep gloating over your jumbo-sized, mutated brains that discovered penicillin and rat poison and anti-malarial drugs and in vitro fertilization. Keep smiling defiantly into your sixth, seventh and eighth decades of life and just watch what I have in store for your species."

Dementia is a general, pathological term best described as what happens when the mental qualities that separate humans from other mammals narrows. This means that the fine motor skills, like buttoning a shirt or blouse, become cumbersome or impossible; the ability to recall recent comments (spoken or heard) deteriorates, or is lost; judgment detaches from reason; and language skills regress, to name a few of the debilitations.

While there are a number of relatively uncommon etiologies to **dementia**, I'll start by briefly discussing the **second most common form**, which is **vascular**, and most frequently seen in patients with significant risk factors, which include the familiar high blood pressure, high LDL cholesterol (see section: "CAN DRUGS KEEP MY ARTERIES OPEN? *Mother Nature's nemesis–the statin drugs*"), diabetes, and tobacco use. This form of dementia can present very differently from patient to patient because the pathological process involves areas of the brain damaged by small strokes, originating from progressive accumulation of arteriosclerosis in blood vessels and their eventual clotting (see section: "CAN ASPIRIN SAVE ME FROM A HEART ATTACK OR STROKE? *Aspirin–pissing off Mother Nature*"), with subsequent brain damage dependent on the location of the vessel involved.

So-called *Alzheimer's disease* accounts for probably three-quarters of all cases of dementia. The term Alzheimer's is applied to a more specific form of dementia first described by a German physician of that name who identified a patient in the early 1900s with symptoms of dementia, and whose brain autopsy demonstrated specific microscopic anatomical variations from normal.

Before I superficially touch on these pathological findings (the subject is important enough with aging baby boomers potentially bankrupting Medicare, as it is currently written), let me put our brain capacity into perspective. It's estimated that there are *approximately 100 billion nerve cells* in a normal human brain. These very specialized cells have multiple branches that allow for the potential of somewhere around *one hundred trillion biochemical connections*! As you progress from stomping your fingers on the piano to "Chopsticks," and on to concert-pianist master, you have made ever-increasing connections that allow your graduation from "stop that damn noise" to a standing ovation at Carnegie Hall.

Everything you encounter in your environment, from what you perceive in the womb to that final goodbye (assuming "normal" brain function for your age), makes biochemical connections between *neurons* (brain cells). Every experience, (what you are taught, what you read or hear, your social contacts and the opinions you derive from them, your acquired pleasures or fears), forms a new or altered link in that cornucopia of cells in your head. I would guess that at this point in the discussion, MN's expression is probably neutral. After all, mutations are random (or set in motion by a power she dare not confront) and no fault of her own. Her patience is understandable because she knows that the rest of our DNA, including that portion responsible for the intellectual lottery that we won in our skulls, isn't up to the task of immortality.

So, let's briefly explore the disparity between what we would hope for in our old age and how that sometimes "goes down the tubes." Using the idiom as a segue, there are tubes and then there are *microtubules*. The latter *are numerous dynamic protein structures that align within brain nerve cells and form conduits for the movement of substances necessary for sustaining the life of the cell*. The alignment of these molecular highways is critical to the nerve cell's function.

Special unrelated proteins, (called *tau proteins*) help maintain the orderly positioning of these *microtubules*. Within brain tissue, there is a protein fragment (called *beta-amyloid*), which is normally broken down and eliminated. But in cases of Alzheimer's, this beta-amyloid accumulates and tends to form plaques between nerve cells that inhibit their ability to communicate with each other. Furthermore, these *abnormal plaques biochemically interfere with the normal function of tau proteins, causing them to stick and clump, resulting in a collapse in the orderly positioning of microtubules responsible for the methodical delivery of life-sustaining molecules*, and thus begins the process of nerve-cell destruction.

As these neurons die, the Alzheimer's patient demonstrates progressive changes in his or her mental capabilities, the observed deterioration depending on the location of the damage. There is a portion of the brain (called the *hippocampus*), which is particularly vulnerable to damage and, since it's responsible for short-term memory, forgetfulness of recent events is a common early sign of Alzheimer's.

Now what? As you can imagine, if someone could come up with a cure or, better yet, a preventive, for this "curse," somebody would make a helluva lot of money. And, many drug companies and non-commercial labs are working day and night in search of a breakthrough. Part of the problem is a chicken-or-the-egg dilemma. Are the abnormalities I've described above *causing* the problem, or are they merely the *consequences* of the problem?

By now, MN has probably abandoned her neutral expression and is smiling. She's content that our expanded intellect is unlikely to solve this violation of her natural order. There have been a few stabs in the darkness of our ignorance that have yielded some uncelebrated results. For example, there are unimpressive studies suggesting that Vitamin E (*alpha tocopherol*) may play some positive role (see section: "VITAMINS . . . TOO MUCH OF A GOOD THING? *Voodoo vitamins and other deceptions*"), but I personally remain doubtful for a number of reasons, including my experience with my own patients. In my opinion, the same statement applies for the FDA approved drugs classified as *acetyl cholinesterase inhibiters* and *N-methyl D-aspartate inhibitors*, both of which have effects on neurotransmitters, molecules that play a role in neuron-to-neuron communication. But when you look at the pathology I described above, messing with the communicators seems a bit like treating a rusted door by moving it to a state with a lower humidity.

There are also claims regarding the prophylactic use of certain vitamins and minerals. Vitamin E is singled out again, as well as B6, D, folic acid, B12 and copper. The problem with these assertions is that while no one would argue that these vitamins and minerals are necessary for normal brain function, and that deficiencies might contribute to Alzheimer's, to take the leap that higher than metabolically necessary amounts of these substances can somehow prevent or significantly slow the progression of the disease is unjustified.

So, what the hell are we supposed to do while we wait for that breakthrough that sends a pharmaceutical stock through the ceiling, or hands the Nobel Prize in Medicine to some genius holed up in his dusty lab with his fourteen-year-old cat? Not to mention that annoying simper on MN's face? First of all, *exercise.* A revealing study in a prestigious medical journal (published in 2013) followed more than 19,000 patients, 80% male, for an average of 25 years. Their physical fitness was assessed (by treadmill exercise testing) at baseline. The purpose of the study was to see if the level of fitness in middle age had any predictive value for the development of dementia in later life. They found that the **more physically fit** the participants were in the beginning of the study, the **less** likely they were to develop **any** form of dementia later in life. So, it would seem, as I would expect, "working" our biology in a "natural" way can tip the scales in our favor as our aging DNA looks for an evolutionary excuse to take us down (not physically fit = bad genes and wasted food).

Now, understand that the original mutation that started the process leading to our current brainpower had to represent a survival advantage or it wouldn't have happened. Once we reached a threshold of intelligence that sustained that advantage, anything that followed was no longer **necessarily** an **additional** advantage. Think about it: all we really needed was enough gray matter in our heads to recognize that a sharp rock attached to a stick in the hands of fifty men from the clan could pretty much place us at the top of the food chain. How do the supplementary smarts that provide for motorized vehicles that take us to the drive-up window (through which a 2000 calorie, multi-deck, salty burger is passed) add any extra survival advantage?

Another recent study followed over 93,000 women, ages 50-79, for approximately 8 years. The researchers were looking for any adverse health outcomes in those participants who sat for 10 hours a day or longer (compared to those who sat half as much of the time). *The authors found not only an increase in heart attacks for those who sat longer, but (even more relevant to this section) an increase in strokes. Particularly revealing for me was that even those women who sat for 10 hours or longer, and who also exercised during their non-sitting hours, suffered excess heart attacks and strokes compared to women who sat half the time. The take home here, as I see it, is that sitting (doing nothing physical) is not only detrimental in and of itself, but may actually counter the positive effects of exercise.* No matter how you slice it, it seems inactivity (both physical and mental) screams survival worthlessness to our DNA. What really struck me about this study was its unintended logic. Think about it. How much time (if any) would you guess our earliest biped (walking erect on two legs) predecessor spent sitting? The danger we face is that we lose sight of the fact that our intelligence is not necessarily a guaranteed survival advantage.

I recommend that you do what a normal inquisitive energetic youthful human being should do. Look for, and participate in, *change*. This not only makes new brain connections, but, I suspect, may also suppress the formation of bad stuff between and in our neurons. While repetitious patterns of behavior have their advantages (expecting the berries on the vine when the weather gets warm enough to make the animal skin covering your Neanderthal backside uncomfortable), they have even greater disadvantages when our lives are so complex that in the name of projected success we isolate ourselves, believing that more focused attention in an introverted niche provides us with an advantage. This makes about as much sense as believing that if you adopt a lifestyle in which you sit all day resting your muscles, you'll prime yourself for that great race. So, *meet new people. Engage in new experiences. Develop new skills, both physical and mental. Change your routine*. Because as you follow this advice, I'm betting that *good genes turn on, and bad genes turn off,* and a host of yet-to-be-discovered *hormones* rush into our brains, making sweet, protective new biochemical connections, so that when MN checks the score board of our lives, she's fooled into celebrating our Little League accomplishments, unaware that some of us may still remember eating hot dogs at Ebbets Field and the Polo Grounds.

CAN DRUGS KEEP
MY ARTERIES OPEN?

Mother Nature's nemesis–the statin drugs

Joining the ranks of vernacular terms such as "stomach flu" (usually medically inaccurate, but more socially acceptable than diarrhea or the "runs"), the words high or low cholesterol have become a hallmark synonymous with one's state of health. The average person subjected to the media blitz that touts the health benefits of "low cholesterol" foods may self-deceive into believing those calories count less. In fact, there is speculation that the shift to low-fat, low-cholesterol diets decades ago is partially responsible for a sugar-induced epidemic of obesity. Be that as it may, understanding a simplified version of cholesterol metabolism in the context of our evolutionary journey and our expanded life span tied to human ingenuity is helpful in providing both the motivation for serious consideration for lowering so-called *"bad" cholesterol (LDL)* and a reason why the statin drugs are MN's nemesis.

Cholesterol is essential for human life. This molecule is assembled in our livers and, after a series of biochemical conversions, winds up as ***adrenal*** and ***sex hormones***. These hormones' lineage traced back to cholesterol classifies them as "steroids," related to, but not to be confused with, "prednisone," a man-made derivative frequently used in medicine to treat a variety of conditions involving inflammation.

One such hormone synthesized in the outer portion of our two adrenal glands, each of which sit on top of our two kidneys, is called ***aldosterone***, which instructs our kidneys to conserve water, a necessity when we left oceans of salt water for dry land, the wet stuff now a premium commodity.

Another hormone produced from the cholesterol molecule by the outer portion of our kidneys is ***cortisol***. This is often described as the "***stress hormone***," since it is produced in higher amounts through a complex series of biochemical reactions beginning with our brains' recognition that we are in deep shit. One of the functions of ***cortisol*** is to raise our blood sugar level (countering the effects of insulin, which drives glucose into cells) and at the same time stimulate the liver to manufacture more of the high-energy compound. So, depending on whether we're on a vacation in Hawaii, or running away from a charging pit bull, we can count on the appropriate levels of ***cortisol*** to keep things in balance.

In addition to ***aldosterone*** and ***cortisol***, small amounts of ***sex hormones*** are also derived from the cholesterol molecule and manufactured in the outer portion of our adrenal glands. A much greater quantity of sex hormones of cholesterol origin (for example, ***progesterone***, ***testosterone*** and ***estradiol***) is produced in the sex organs.

And finally, and most ubiquitously, ***the cholesterol molecule is essential to the integrity of every cell in our bodies, playing a critical role in the structure that defines the "envelope" (or cell membrane), responsible for letting the good things in and the bad things out***. In summary: No cholesterol, no life!

So why then does cholesterol carry the potential to kill us? While this seems a pretty straightforward question, the answer is complex enough to make *lipidologists* (physicians who specialize in all aspects of cholesterol metabolism and its potential pathological impact) nearly as rare as twelve-year-olds with college degrees. My job here is to ignore MN's really nasty glare and present only the necessary information that I feel is important in helping you make a decision regarding possible therapy with a *statin* drug, even if you have been told that your cholesterol levels are not bad or even "okay".

Bear with me. Cholesterol by itself won't dissolve in water. So how the heck does it get around in our bodies? When cholesterol is manufactured in the liver it must be packaged in a way that makes it soluble in our blood. This is accomplished by wrapping it up in a parcel (the combination of cholesterol and its covering is referred to as a *lipoprotein*), which can carry its core freely to various destinations served by our blood vessels. Depending on the make-up of the lipoproteins (the wrapping), lipidologists classify the packages in five different ways. Please stay awake; it will pay off!

I'll start with one of these packages, which I wish could be labeled Package #1, but unfortunately it's called a *chylomicron* (sorry). This guy actually has very little cholesterol in its core, but is loaded with something called *triglycerides*, which you may recall having been mentioned by your physician when discussing your blood work. These triglycerides are made up of a molecule that hooks up with *three fatty acids* (these fatty acids are best thought of as fat such as *unsaturated*, *monosaturated*, *polyunsaturated*, the evil *trans fat*, and the good guys or *omegas*). These chylomicrons form as you digest fat and then move the product from the inside of your small intestine, through its wall and are finally shuttled into channels (called *lymphatics*). These channels, which carry the chylomicrons, eventually empty into your *heart* and get distributed into your circulation, releasing their triglycerides as their fatty acid components, which are supercharged with energy [more so than even glucose (sugar)] to the delight of such high-octane users as heart and skeletal muscle.

Now to what I wish we might call Package #2, which is abbreviated **VLDL (Very Low Density Lipoprotein)** in defiance of more palatable simplicity for the non-scientist. This guy (VLDL), with its own special casing, also contains triglycerides and its attached fatty acids. This package works its way to the tiny blood vessels in fat and muscle and then turns over its payload of triglycerides (its fatty acids), the remaining leftover lipoprotein is our Package #3, which is abbreviated as **IDL (Intermediate Density Lipoprotein)**.

Okay, now we get down to business. The IDL is then either sent back to the liver or is further degraded through a series of steps (that for our purposes is about as important as the take-home revelations about life from the latest reality show) into our Package #4, the infamous **LDL (Low Density Lipoprotein)** or **"bad" cholesterol**. This LDL or "bad" cholesterol particle carries triglycerides, but is the main transporter of cholesterol in our bodies and is welcomed by our cells, which bind it and use it to maintain the integrity of their **cell membranes**, those envelopes surrounding the contents of every cell. Containing a higher concentration of cholesterol, some of these LDL particles are **smaller and denser than others**. These little buggers can overwhelm the cell (as they are picked up by special molecular **receptors** on cell membranes – including liver cells) and thus are capable of causing excess deposition of cholesterol in arteries. In addition, these smaller and denser LDL particles have the particularly pronounced ability to **incite an inflammatory process** in the delicate single-cell lining of blood vessels (called **endothelium**), which is particularly dangerous in initiating and advancing the process of hardening of the arteries or **atherosclerosis** (more later).

A brief comment on different ways of measuring LDL is in order with growing evidence that the **number** of **LDL particles** (or **LDL-P**) may represent a more accurate assessment of cardiovascular risk than the standard LDL (or more specifically the LDL-C, which we've been discussing so far). The LDL-C (the standard measurement) represents the ***amount or concentration of cholesterol in LDL particles***, and since there is variation in concentration from particle to particle the LDL-C is in essence an estimate. Now (before you say: "What the hell? My damn cardiologist might just as well bring out the leaches if he's been altering my dose of statins based on some outdated measurement!"), it should be made clear that LDL-C has served the general public extraordinarily well for decades. Dosage adjustments of statin drugs based on LDL-C values have saved many lives and greatly improved quality of life for multitudes of patients who would have otherwise succumbed to heart attack and/or stroke. In many cases statin therapy effectively lowers ***both*** LDL-C ***and*** LDL-P. If triglycerides are high (as mentioned earlier, the LDL particle also carries triglycerides), there may be less available "room" in a given LDL particle, which may result in the biologically necessity of cranking out a higher ***number*** of LDL particles to accommodate the cholesterol that couldn't find an "unrented apartment." There are circumstances where a drug may reduce the LDL-C and have less effect on the LDL-P. The opposite can also be true.

The take home here? Based solely on LDL-C measurements, some patients may be either ***over*** or ***under*** treated with statin drugs. Controversy remains, but for now (until more work is done and the LDL-P test becomes more readily available), let me reiterate that in my practice over decades (both before and after the availability of statin drugs and the evidence-based clinical results demonstrating their value), ***using the LDL-C for guidance has made a remarkably positive impact on the length and quality of life in the thousands of patients I've treated with documented vascular disease.***

Finally, to the #5 package, the ***HDL (High Density Lipoprotein)***, or the "good" cholesterol. While the true value of this "savior" in potentially reducing the risk of vascular disease (primarily heart attack and stroke) has recently come under some fire, its biochemistry would seem to mitigate the criticism. This having been said, in my own experience, I have seen a significant number of heart attacks in women with very high HDLs (more later). This proposed good-guy (or gal) lipoprotein begins its retrieval journey in the liver and intestine, from which its incomplete form is released. "Junior" HDL will mature into the smallest and densest of our five packages. It travels to various tissues and picks up cholesterol from the cell and transports it back to the liver where it's removed from our circulation by special *receptors.*

Alright, we're ready to take the boards in Lipidology. And except for our defaming comments about LDL, MN has sat back and listened, nodding her head as the approving matriarch of the evolutionary process that was the basis for much of what we explained. When she heard our comments about "bad" cholesterol, however, I suspect she toyed with a more irritated countenance. "LDL is one of my innocent children. It would mean you no harm if you just died when you were supposed to." Her comment begs the question: "Since no mammals in nature, possessing a similar lipid metabolism, die from heart attacks or strokes, what the hell did we do to screw things up so royally?" And also: "If we're so damn smart, can we do something about it?"

First, let's speak to the obvious: the longer you live (especially when your species' intelligence exploded with "tricks" to combat your natural enemies, be they microscopic or behemoth), the older your DNA, the more likely it will mutate. This is a biological fact and not much different than what you would logically expect if a complicated machine with many moving parts is kept busy continuously. Even with maintenance, something, sooner or later, will malfunction. Depending on the biological consequences of those mutations you will either benefit or suffer. Keener vision or hearing is a good thing, having only one eye or one ear is a bad thing. Adverse consequences of mutated DNA need not be immediately evident. So let's look at an extreme case to make two crucial points.

There is an inherited disease of cholesterol metabolism called *familial hypercholesterolemia*. These patients, who have inherited only one bad gene from a single parent who carries it (note that an even worse case occurs if two bad genes are inherited) have a significant reduction in the receptors that accept cholesterol from HDL ("good" cholesterol) as it returns its payload to the liver. The result is a very high LDL ("bad" cholesterol) in their blood. Remember, if the number of receptors in the liver that ordinarily "take" the cholesterol "plucked" out of cells (the job of HDL) are reduced, the cholesterol has no place to go except back into your blood. Think of a garbage truck that picks up a load from your house and finds that the landfill is "closed," so it takes the load back to your house and dumps it on the street.

Patients with familial hypercholesterolemia are prone to premature heart attacks and/or strokes not uncommonly seen by age 30 or 40. Now, think about it. Even though we see an obviously premature (by modern medical standards) adverse health event, the abnormality was present at conception. He or she will probably live long enough to reproduce and pass the bad gene to offspring. So, the two points illustrated here are *1) even with a really lousy gene, humans can live long enough to introduce it, or add it, to the gene pool and 2) genetics play a critical role in determining the configuration and quantity of every substance and reaction described in our very simplified earlier discussion about the five lipoprotein packages and their function.*

There are many possible mutations far subtler than familial hypercholesterolemia, which can "hide" in our DNA for generations; this creeping crud of adverse coding (along with lifestyle indiscretions) has the potential to negatively impact our blood vessels and introduce pathological outcomes not seen in the non-human natural environment. (I can see MN nodding: "You bet your ass, Dr. Boy!") When normally functioning, elaborate biochemical interactions with uncanny balance are assaulted with an inappropriate diet or lack of physical exercise (or just a lousy draw from the grab bag of adversely mutated genes), it doesn't take much to gum up MN's machinery.

Let's get just a bit more specific and focus on triglycerides, LDL and HDL, and finally address the incredibly important role of the statin drugs.

How do high *triglycerides* make trouble for us? First of all, most studies suggest the damage to vessel walls is not a direct effect of triglycerides, but rather the consequences of "down-the-road" effects. For purposes of this discussion (and with the hope of keeping your eyes open), I'll condense decades of articles and speculations on the bad things excess triglycerides do to our arteries into the simplest of statements: while the value of real estate is often determined by location, location, location, triglycerides probably do most of their mischief through *inflammation, inflammation, inflammation.* (See section: "HAS MY BODY TURNED AGAINST ME? *Inflammation – overdoing a good thing*"). A really high-fat meal actually *turns on genes* that produce substances that result in inflammation. High triglycerides can have an adverse effect on the level of HDL ("good" cholesterol) and negatively impact certain proposed anti-inflammatory characteristics of the good stuff. Large amounts of fatty acids released by high levels of triglycerides (remember – triglycerides carry three attached fatty acids) predispose the lining of blood vessels (remember, the cells are called *endothelium*) to an inflammatory process. And finally, even the protein in cells that transport fatty acids under certain conditions may play a role in inflammation. So, there you have it: inflammation, inflammation, inflammation! More later.

Now to how excess LDL ("bad" cholesterol) in our blood harms us, with deliberate omission of the LDL-C/LDL-P issues addressed earlier. It's important to remember that some LDL in its native form is part of normal lipid chemistry as it carries the majority of cholesterol in our blood as a precursor to the formation of certain hormones in various organs and provides a critical component of the *cell membrane* (the envelope of cells that hold them together as we discussed earlier) that must allow certain molecules in and others out. So what goes wrong?

Back to the tidy balance that MN has instilled in every aspect of a normally functioning organism. *Molecules* (assembled from atoms) possess the capability of interacting with other molecules or atoms. So, as we discussed earlier (see section: "VITAMINS . . . TOO MUCH OF A GOOD THING? *Voodoo vitamins and other deceptions*") in this soup (our blood) of potential interactions, including atoms or groups of atoms with a certain characteristic that can react with the *oxygen* (remember, the process is called *oxidation*) and form very unstable substances (remember *free radicals?*), which, if not counteracted by *antioxidants*, which MN has supplied in ample quantities, can get into a cell (such as the *endothelium* – the lining of blood vessels) and screw things up with yet another inflammatory process. This detrimental process not only does damage directly, but also attracts cells that don't belong in a normal blood vessel lining, triggering the release of a variety of substances from them that eventually turns a smooth, normal blood vessel lining into one that sports a plaque. This plaque can progress into something thicker that restricts the diameter of the vessel until all that crap finally ruptures through into the remaining restricted opening and a high percentage blockage invites a *blood clot* and a 911 call.

So you see, if our LDL is low enough, MN can handle it with her complementary antioxidants. But sit on our assess, make soda and candy a staple in our diet, or just be unlucky enough to have inherited enough crappy genes to send your LDL number to a level you wished represented your bank account, and MN says: "You blew it, Bozo, so please die, especially if you're still young enough to have kids."

Finally, (no applause, please) I'll finish with *HDL*, the "good" cholesterol. About three quarters of the protein content in the outer covering of our package #5 lipoprotein (HDL) is a special complex molecule that chemically grabs cholesterol wherever it can find it. This can occur both in our circulation and from within cells. So, let me repeat what I said earlier and expand the discussion just a little (I have my reasons): **HDL** acts like a hungry scavenger that carries its payload back to the liver (so-called *reverse cholesterol transport*). Now once back in the liver this newly "dumped" cholesterol winds up in our bile (the stuff made in the liver as a detergent to break up fats in preparation for their absorption through our small intestine and eventually into our circulation). This process is accomplished in two ways.

The first is by liver cells (called *hepatocytes*), which take the cholesterol and channel it directly into the bile.

The second method involves *a special protein that pulls the cholesterol out of the HDL and transfers it to LDL*, which is then dumped into our bile. This special protein involved in the second method just described has a really nasty name that I will just call **CETP.** Why am I bothering with this? It's because in our species, ingenuity (not to mention the financial motivations of drug companies) often sparks research. And early research revealed that *if you blocked this CEPT guy, HDL went way up and LDL went way down*! Terrific result.

So, clinical studies using agents that blocked CEPT proceeded, and great cholesterol numbers where seen in the blood tests from lots of patients and, with great anticipation, everyone (including Wall Street investors) waited for clinical results, which really begs the question: "Do these terrific numbers translate in the real world of patients into a reduction in heart attacks and strokes? Guess what? *It was a complete bust!* If MN had a middle finger, it would be raised at full mast. Take home message: *it's not just the reduction in numbers that matters; it's how and by what mechanism you achieve a reduction in LDL*. Why am I emphasizing this point? Because it sings the praises of the statin drugs even louder as you will soon realize.

Alright, let's get to it. The statin drugs: *MEVACOR* (Lovastatin), *PRAVACHOL* (Pravastatin), *ZOCOR* (Simvastatin), *LESCOL* (Fluvastatin), *LIPITOR* (Atovastatin), *CRESTOR* (Rosuvastin) and *LIVALO* (Pitavastatin). How do they work? While a diet high in cholesterol can contribute to higher blood levels, most cholesterol in our bodies is manufactured in the liver. As in any biochemical progression leading to a finished product, basic smaller molecular units are joined through the actions of special proteins (*enzymes*), which facilitate the process. One crucial enzyme in the process leading to the production of cholesterol molecules in the liver has a designation that probably helps explain why lipidology lectures put more aspiring medical students to sleep than warm milk. The enzyme is called *HMG-CoA Reductase* (told ya). So, what statins do, is they *inhibit this important enzyme in the synthesis of cholesterol* and (among other good things, such as a tendency to lower triglycerides and raise HDL) in doing so, *substantially drop the amount of the "bad" cholesterol (LDL) in our blood*. Now this brings to mind my earlier discussion regarding the very promising reductions in blood levels of LDL with CEPT blocking agents (remember, it was shown that these agents really knocked the socks off of LDL and soared the HDL with *no* clinical benefit). Well, the story is very different here with the statins.

The first statin (*Lovastatin* – later branded as *Mevacor*) was discovered in 1978. But it wasn't approved for release as a therapy for high cholesterol until the late 1980s. As of today, various statin drugs have been tested in hundreds of thousands (if not more) of patients worldwide.

I'll start with the negative: in very rare circumstances (estimated at about 0.44 per 10,000 patients, or one patient in more than 20,000) severe muscle damage (*rhabdomyolysis*) can occur resulting in kidney failure; statistically, with long-term therapy, there is about a 9% greater chance of developing diabetes than if you weren't taking a statin; somewhere between 10-15 % of patients taking statin drugs may experience some form of ***muscle pain or weakness***, which may be related to a genetic predisposition (in my experience with older patient populations their reported adverse effects are often related to arthritic issues and when the drug is stopped, there is often no improvement in symptoms); and finally, ***elevations of liver enzymes*** in 1 to 3%, which are often mild and almost always easily reversible by withholding the drug.

So, what's so good about statins? Why take them and why are they MN's nemesis? First of all, ***one study after another has demonstrated substantial reductions in heart attacks and strokes***. Even if other risk factors [such as high blood pressure, diabetes, sedentary lifestyle (with or without obesity), family history of vascular disease] don't exist, the bad vascular outcomes in patients with high LDL cholesterol, in particular, are significantly reduced. ***The magic of the statins seems to work both by lowering LDL and countering inflammation in the cells that line our blood vessels***. As we discussed earlier, inflammation is an integral part of the dirty tricks played on us by elevated triglycerides and high LDL.

Recently, after years of scrutinizing the vast body of medical literature, the American Heart Association and the American College of Cardiology presented new guidelines for the use of statin drugs in the prevention and treatment of vascular disease in a number of patient populations. One general suggestion was for the practitioner to assess a patient's ***risk*** for vascular disease based on more than just the level of LDL in blood. This suggestion has prompted some criticism, the detractors emphasizing that the proposal will vastly expand statin use. Personally, I think both the recommendation and the criticism are naïve. Since when in medicine do we ignore the total patient, focusing on an isolated symptom or finding?

Other recommendations by the panel of experts include automatically treating anyone with known vascular disease or anyone with an LDL of 190 mg/dL or greater (generally levels of ***100 to***

129 are considered pretty damn close to "just fine," but for me, in anyone, I want to see them *below 100*).

Additional statin treatment recommendations include anyone with Type II diabetes (the type that usually doesn't require insulin and is related to unhealthy diet and inactivity), and finally, anyone between the ages of 40 and 75 who, based on a formula provided, have a 10-year risk of developing vascular disease of 7.5% or more, which incidentally would qualify *any male 65 or older*, since death in that gender and age group is usually not the result of being struck by a meteor.

Okay, so these learned bodies of highly respected individuals with impeccable credentials have released their guidelines. For me, they're okay, but why even a hint of dissatisfaction? Because I honestly believe, after decades of experience with thousands of patients with vascular disease who I follow on a regular basis, that their recommendations don't go far enough! I would suggest that *any male over the age of forty and any female over the age of fifty*, with no contraindication, should take a statin drug for life, so long as they do not develop legitimate adverse side effects such as significant muscle pain or weakness and/or a significant rise in liver enzymes. And *the dose taken need not be as high as is recommended by the new guidelines*. These guidelines appropriately reflect the medical literature, which tends to employ high rather than low doses of a drug under consideration to both encourage the elucidation of its positive effects and any potential adverse consequences. So, as the criticism occasionally flows in from a few of my colleagues who accuse me of being overly aggressive, I might ask them to speculate on the state of the Medicare trust fund if every 21-year-old since 1940 (statins were not available then) was required to take a low dose of the drug.

While it is probably true, and unfortunate, that there would likely have been a relatively small number of *rhabdomyolysis* cases (with great consequence to those individuals and their families), and probably a fair number of patients with ***reversible liver damage,*** even if we assume a worse-case scenario, millions of Americans would not have had their heart attack or stroke, many of them surviving and (if we could exclude Alzheimer's) nursing homes today might be offering two-for-one deals to try and fill their vacancies. Medicare would be swimming in cash, the government trying (and no doubt finding a way) to move the money elsewhere, and generic statins would be sitting on the over-the-counter shelves next to vitamins.

So here we are – a species whose cerebral mutations gave us an unfair advantage over the rest of the natural world. And what did we do? The reproductively active found ways to minimize the adverse impact of crappy genes and passed them on. Many of the older within the species reveled in the creation of machines that did their work and a growing number of individuals got fat and lazy. ***But, more optimistically, and in further defiance of natural selection, we discovered a class of drugs (the statins) that prevented, or stopped, or reversed one of the consequences MN had counted on for punishment for our biological sins***.

She could never have guessed that our species could, or would, be capable of creating yet another nemesis for her after the discovery of statins. Dare I whisper that a compound is currently undergoing clinical trials that blocks a protein called ***PCSK9***, which plays an important role in ***deactivating receptor sites*** on the surface of liver cells that remove LDL? ***Blocking this protein increases the receptors' ability to function, resulting in an impressive drop in LDL***. And recent data reveals that the drug, injected under the skin every two weeks, also has <u>no</u> apparent adverse effects on glucose metabolism, which means there is probably no additional risk for developing diabetes.

I see MN turning towards me with an expression that appears less than pleased. "Say what?"

IS BOOZE BAD?

Alcohol—one of Mother Nature's best friends

Let's start with a brief fictitious story. About 2 ½ million years ago, an ape-like creature, pretty well-adapted to standing on two feet, but no Fred Astaire, was unaware of a mutation in one of his sperm cells or her ovarian cells. Either, or both, of those modified cells produced twin offspring (male and female) who were both just a little smarter than other youths in this ancient community. The twins had learned that when the daylight lasted just so long and the temperature was just so warm, berries on a vine about a mile away were ripe. So, each year at the same time, the twins secretly made the journey, picked the berries, ate a few and hid the others from the rest of the tribe.

One year, after a bumper crop of berries, the twins headed home with handfuls (maybe primitive bagfuls if they were smart enough) of the delicacy. Upon arriving back at the community just before sunrise, our enlightened protagonists grew concerned that they might be discovered with their stash as a few of their tribesmen stirred in their sleep. Panicky, they looked for places to hide their berries for later consumption. Finding a naturally hollowed

out basin in a large boulder, our smarter-than-the-average con-
noisseurs quickly dumped the berries into the basin. The fruit
still not adequately hidden, they found a nearby large flat rock,
smeared on a coating of wet mud and applied the result as a cover,
hiding their culinary treasure. Then, try as they might, for many
days there never seemed a safe opportunity to uncover and enjoy
their bonanza.

Later, the men went on a hunting expedition and the women
on a distant gathering mission. Our quiz kids feigned an illness
and stayed behind. The opportunity ripe (not as ripe as the long-
stored berries), our malingerers raided their stash. To their dis-
may, the berries didn't taste exactly as they had remembered. But
the recollection of their heroic effort and their appetite for the
fruit overpowered our twins and they ate every berry and even the
acrid liquid left behind.

Near sunset, the hunters approached their encampment and
found the women who had returned earlier from their gathering
responsibilities shaking with fear. You see, our twins were inappropriately laughing, stumbling, crying and even making gestures
that either made no sense or were off-limits even for a primitive
people. Unevolved as these hunters were, they nevertheless feared
unseen evil forces and demons that they believed inhabited their
world. So, it's no surprise that our berry hoarders were promptly
killed, their bodies burned and their ashes secretly scattered over
the land of a competing tribe. Don't you just love stories with hap-
py endings?

So, what's the lesson in this? ***When fruit is placed in an environment with little or no oxygen, the yeast that is present converts the sugar
in the fruit to obtain energy for cellular function, leaving ethanol (alcohol) and carbon dioxide as waste products.*** True, but not exactly the
main point. How about, don't drink and drive because you might
kill someone including yourself? Absolutely true, but that's not all.
Perhaps, despite what you've read (and embraced with self-serving,

and I would suspect, self-deceiving vigor), my story might suggest that I'm not a big fan of alcohol, based on my medical reading and my experience with patients? Bingo!

Let's begin by revisiting the story I just invented. In actuality, a similar scenario probably did take place near the dawn of our species. And ever since those alcohol-induced effects were experienced, *Homo sapiens* were off and running with creative ways to distill an alcohol-containing product into ever higher concentrations of what can be referred to (with a little literary license) as yeast and bacteria pee and poop.

So, what about all those stories in newspapers and on TV, and even in the scientific journals, that tout the benefits of alcohol in moderation, including proposed benefits in reducing coronary artery disease? *If you read these studies carefully and pay particular attention to how they were designed and the methods used, you will find that any positive conclusions claimed are all flawed!*

One misconception that seems to have legs is that the French, who consume lots of fat and also lots of alcohol, have an impressively low rate of coronary artery disease. A clue to the truth can be gleaned from their obesity rates. Relative to other highly industrialized countries, France is low on the list. So, if they're eating all this high-calorie fat and significantly caloric-rich booze, how come they're not running to the bariatric surgeon for gastric bypass surgery (see section: "WHAT'S THE DEAL WITH BARIATRIC SURGERY? *Evolutionary impatience*"). At least part of the story is their gene pool (ignoring the make-up of the genetic characteristics of recent immigrant populations). When you study a biological process as complex as vascular disease, it seems absurd to so grossly simplify it with a statistical analysis rather than with large-population prospective studies, which in the case of the claims made about the French population, would be logistically impossible to construct. Suggesting a meaningful relationship exists between French consumption of fat and alcohol and the low incidence of coronary artery disease is like proposing a cause and effect relationship between the wearing of kilts or the playing of bag pipes and the incidence of acne in Scottish youth.

Okay, now let's look at the chemical itself. From a human standpoint, alcohol is an **unnatural toxin**. It's broken down in the body through two major enzyme-driven steps that take place in the liver. The first of which briefly converts the alcohol to an even more toxic substance (**acetaldehyde**), which is highly damaging to every cell in the body through its adverse effects on the **microtubules** that ferry proteins and other critical substances from one part of the cell to another (see section: "HOW DO I KEEP MY BRAIN YOUNG? **Dementia/Alzheimer's – Mother Nature's revenge**"). It seems reasonable that such inherently destructive biology could explain **the association of alcohol to cancer of the mouth, throat, voice box and esophagus**. Acetaldehyde is quickly acted upon by another enzyme, which alters its structure into a somewhat less-toxic substance (**an acetate**).

Let's start with the extreme and then apply some logic here. The adverse effects of excess amounts of alcohol read like the winning lottery numbers in MN's playbook.

The **liver** can work only so hard for so long. Eventually, the damage from alcohol is so extensive that hepatic cells (liver cells, or **hepatocytes**) can no longer keep up and scarring occurs. As the liver shrinks in size and function, (called **cirrhosis**), the vein draining all the blood returning to the liver for detoxification on the way back to the heart from the gastrointestinal tract (the **portal vein**) is subjected to higher and higher pressures. Eventually, the backflow will cause enormous swelling in the abdominal cavity, the legs and, in men, the scrotum. In my training, I saw the scrotums of newly diagnosed cirrhotic patients the size of cantaloupes.

Nerve cells in the brain can be permanently damaged by alcohol. Early on, the part of the brain that is responsible for recent memory (we alluded to this structure, called the **hippocampus**, in the section: "HOW CAN I KEEP MY BRAIN YOUNG? ***Dementia/ Alzheimer's – Mother Nature's revenge***") is particularly sensitive to alcohol. In patients with cirrhosis, the liver may be incapable of detoxifying various products from intestinal bacteria; the result is altered consciousness, usually progressive drowsiness and, if un-treated, coma and death.

The ***pancreas*** can become inflamed with excess alcohol and, in an acute phase, exquisitely painful. Long term, the pancreas is predisposed to developing cancer, which is often hidden from a patient until the disease process is far advanced.

The ***stomach*** is irritated by alcohol and increases its production of acid, which can lead to erosions and bleeding.

The ***kidneys,*** like any organ, can be adversely affected by alco-hol. While the changes are often less clinically obvious (especially if there isn't concomitant liver disease, which has its own adverse consequences for kidney function), alcohol drastically affects the delicate fluid balance monitored by our kidneys (can you imagine if bars didn't have rest rooms?).

The cells lining our ***lungs*** are also susceptible to damage from alcohol. Patients presenting with unrelated lung problems, such as lung trauma or pneumonia, clinically don't do as well as non-drinkers, when all other factors are taken into consideration.

And now to my specialty. Yes, the heart is also susceptible to the toxic effects of alcohol. Over the years, I have seen a number of cases in which the patient's heart is markedly enlarged and the function substantially reduced. While there are many reasons for this presentation, it is not unusual (after coronary artery disease, valvular abnormalities, metabolic disorders and recent systemic in-fections are excluded) to elicit a history of either current or remote alcohol abuse. Many of these patients may demonstrate abnormali-ties in their heart rhythms, not infrequently, delays in the elec-trical system, or ***atrial fibrillation*** (it's an irregular heart rhythm generated as the result of chaotic electrical activity in the upper chambers of the heart – see section: "WHAT'S THAT FLUTTER IN MY CHEST? *Atrial fibrillation – a valentine from Mother Nature*"). With cessation of alcohol, and not infrequently additional therapy, many of these patients will stabilize or improve.

Alright, so a non-drinker with a medical degree is trying to scare the tar out of his readers who have that occasional, to a-little-more-than occasional, to daily, to the "I'm-too-damn-hung-over-to-read-this-stuff," drink. I won't deny my negative position on alcohol. So then, you might ask: "Why doc are you so bent on this worst-case scenario?" The reason is that *the enzymes responsible for the metabolism of alcohol are dependent on complex genetic factors that determine the amount of, and effectiveness of, these critical substances.* We all know the high variability of an individual's response to alcohol intake. One person may consume huge amounts and demonstrate minimal changes in countenance and behavior. Others eat a rum ball and are under the table. But guess what? What is obvious to any onlooker has nothing whatsoever to do with that individual's cellular response to alcohol. ***You can't see, or feel, those critical life-sustaining microtubules in every damn cell in your body, and you sure as hell can't easily measure the immediate and long-term effects of alcohol on them.*** So, why take a chance with toxic stuff you know might hurt you? *Recommendation: drink no alcohol, unless you're celebrating something so special that you're willing to take a small risk of doing some unseen damage.*

I see MN raising her metaphoric glass filled with pre-human evolutionary reality: "Drink to this. Please!"

WHY CAN'T I LOSE WEIGHT?

Obesity and leptin–the human screw-up

When was the last time you watched one of those nature shows on TV and saw a fat animal struggling in its response to a predator, as much because it was reluctant to stop eating as it was because of its large bulk? The answer is *never*, because in the natural world there are no obese animals.

Let's follow one of these sleek creatures (who will never need a personal trainer, never buy a DVD guaranteeing weight loss, never buy pre-packaged food, never get dizzy with circuit training and never purchase a pill, a supplement, or some powdered leaf with unknown biological consequences) in its daily activities from an unusual perspective, emphasizing what goes on *inside* of it.

Okay, so this fictitious mammal (let's keep it in the family) is a member of a small communal group that roams our mysterious natural environment that's part plains and part jungle, where food and water is scarce one moment and plentiful the next. It's night-time and our animal is sound asleep.

Now let's go *internal* and visit the perfectly proportioned (relative to body size) amount of fat (*adipose tissue*) stored under its hide and around its internal organs. This tissue is composed of individual cells called ***adipocytes, connective tissue*** (something has to hold it together) and ***tiny blood vessels***. These fat cells are "smart" enough to "know" that our animal friend is asleep and in this "knowledge," granted by evolution, ***increases*** a substance it had made and released in ***lower amounts while the animal was awake***. This special "stuff" is a ***peptide*** hormone (a bunch of amino acids linked together) called ***leptin***. Yes, fat is not just for storage; it makes ***hormones*** and is more accurately a gland (an ***endocrine gland,*** to be exact) and not just a love handle or a muffin top.

Leptin at any concentration in the animal's blood traverses special small blood vessels that restrict certain other substances from entering the spinal fluid (these specialized vessels create what is known as the ***blood-brain barrier***) on the way to the brain. The higher concentration of leptin during the night had no problem crossing this barrier on its way to a part of the brain called the ***hypothalamus*** (sorry), which is sort of a mission control over the functions of hormones and their various "assignments" in the nervous system and other parts of the body. ***Leptin reduces the desire to eat***, which is appropriate at dusk since it wouldn't be to our creature's advantage to be searching for the nearest pizzeria in the middle of the night.

So, while our animal sleeps, there are other organs that are "aware" of its slumber, mainly its ***stomach***, but also, to a lesser extent, the upper two sections of its small intestine, the ***duodenum*** and ***jejunum***. These organs' "knowledge" of the sleeping state causes them to modify their production of another hormone called ***ghrelin***. This hormone is regulated ***down*** during the night because one of its jobs is to ***stimulate*** appetite. ***So, need to sleep and not eat – leptin up and ghrelin down.*** Just like leptin, ghrelin easily crosses the blood-brain barrier and gets to the hypothalamus, which shuts down hunger. Interestingly, these two hormones work on the same cells in the hypothalamus, but react with different ***receptors***. (***We've*** *mentioned receptors in other sections, and, by review, it's best to understand them if you picture a door with multiple keyholes, some take the same key, others don't. So, what we have here in this case is that leptin (one type of key) finds its way to our door, inserts itself into a number of keyholes that it fits and then turns, resulting not in an opened door, but rather the triggering of its special effects in the body. The ghrelin "keys" do the same, resulting in their own special effects).*

Now let's **awaken** our animal. Our "smart" stomach and "smart" fat cells know it. Their response? *Fat cells cut back on production of leptin*, blood levels drop, releasing the "brake" on appetite. *Stomach cells make more ghrelin*, blood levels rise and appetite is stimulated. But there's more going on here. Leptin does more things than just depressing desire to eat; it's overwhelmed by a "responsibility" to MN to maintain the ideal balance between energy expenditure and what's left in the tank (fat).

An analogy to clarify: Top off the gas tank in your car, contrary to what is recommended for safety reasons, and your ecologically "smart" car revs up your engine, forcing you to drive faster, no matter what the heck your foot does on the gas pedal, until the excess gas burns off. So, *leptin has many effects*, in addition to appetite suppression, many of which encourage calorie burn at the expense of fat.

Now let's check out what *ghrelin does in addition to stimulating appetite.* One logical effect for an appetite-stimulating hormone is that it increases both your stomach's production of *acid* and its *motility*. Example: your critical response to a question asked during an interview for that once-in-a-lifetime job opportunity is drowned out by your stomach's growling – blame ghrelin. Following in the biochemical footsteps of leptin, and equally devoted to fulfilling MN's demands, ghrelin does other things too, that are designed to address the other end of the spectrum of maintaining weight balance. So, while stimulating you to eat for "fear" that the gas tank in our metaphoric car is too low, it also makes you go slower, no matter what your foot does on the gas pedal, to conserve energy (fat) until you've eaten enough to satisfy MN that you're in balance again. ***Ghrelin does this by increasing your appetite for fats, slowing down your metabolic rate, using more carbs than fat to produce needed energy for body function and even predisposing you towards less physical activity.*** Wow! You must admit that MN is one smart bitch. At the risk of adding confusion to the picture, I can't resist a brief comment regarding research that suggests ghrelin affects another part of our brains (in addition to the hypothalamus), which is responsible for such things as anxiety, sexual desire, motivation and addictive behavior. Maybe next book.

Back to our animal. It's shaken off the cobwebs of sleep. MN's magic is working perfectly in this sleek, fat-balanced creature. On cue, it's hungry.

So our animal searches for food. It gets very lucky and finds a smorgasbord of goodies (food availability in our fictitious land is more often a crap shoot than a done deal). Our animal stuffs itself and then stops eating. The period of time between hunger and feeling full is too short for fat cells to react, crank out more leptin and get it to the brain. Ghrelin will drop, but the physiological effects will take a while. ***So, what stops our animal from eating too much the instant it's full?*** MN has provided another type of cell, also located in our small intestines, primarily in the ***duodenum***, the first portion into which the stomach empties, which produces and secretes its own hormone called ***cholecystokinin*** or ***CCK***. This molecule is another ***peptide***, like many other hormones, and has a number of functions that assist in digestion and neatly tells our animal to stop eating. More specifically, cholecystokinin causes our ***gall bladder*** to contract, which results in a surge of ***bile*** to enter our small bowel, assisting in the digestion of fats in preparation for their absorption into our blood. In addition, CCK stimulates our ***pancreas*** to increase its production and delivery of its own powerful enzymes, which help digest fats, proteins and carbohydrates.

It's a bit controversial, but it seems that the "turn-off" of appetite may be accomplished by two additional effects of CCK, which include the slowing down of stomach emptying (you feel full) and also a direct effect on the *hypothalamus* (similar to leptin's effect in reducing hunger, but accomplishing it more immediately than the more protracted process that originates in fat cells).

So then in summary: *hungry*? Well then, *leptin and CCK are low and ghrelin is high.* Leptin and ghrelin are most applicable over the long haul and CCK more immediate. *No lingering interest in what's still sitting on the all-you-can-eat buffet? Leptin and CCK are both high and ghrelin is low.* This synopsis is accurate, that is, if you are an animal in the wild subjected to what your DNA is programmed to do in the context of natural selection. In all fairness, it's also applicable to an active human being of ideal body weight.

Let's abandon our fictitious, perfectly fit (for many of us struggling with salads, perfectly annoying) animal and move on to us, *people*. About 35% of our species carry that aggravating label of *obesity* and many more – looking at weight tables for "normal" weights based on height, one might think were written by anorexics – the designation of *overweight*, big-boned claims aside. Let's also put aside, for now, CCK and ghrelin.

In many obese patients leptin is chronically <u>ELEVATED</u>. So, what's the problem? *Leptin is an appetite turn-off. High leptin = less eating = energy burn = supermodel. Here's the problem: the damn thing doesn't work! Your leptin levels are through the ceiling and your ravaging through the refrigerator hunting for leftovers or speeding towards fast food. So what the hell is happening here?* And MN, wipe that smirk off your face!

There are a number of possibilities to explain this mess. But first of all, let's get back to the essence of what seems behind all the issues I've raised in this book. If you mutate a brain capable of basic survival into one capable of spitting in the eye of natural selection, not to mention figuring out how to build a nuclear weapon, you're looking for trouble with MN. *We carry 23 pairs of chromosomes that code for about 25,000 specific proteins, but that accounts for only about 2% of our DNA. The remaining 98% doesn't code for a particular protein.* So just what's going on with all this, non-protein producing genetic material? How much of it is senseless and how much of it is responsible for functions unrelated to proteins? *While much is still unknown, you can bet that this vast amount of non-protein producing DNA does plenty.* The point? When you screw with natural selection because you're smart, you probably pay a price for it. When you extend your life by decades, shit happens, not just in the 2% of DNA that codes for protein, but also in the huge remaining 98%. *So, for example, maybe, in some individuals, that nice biologically appropriate high level of Leptin turned out by your fat cells doesn't get across the blood-brain barrier because something in the 98% of non-protein producing DNA (that wouldn't have been there had it not had the luxury of generations of natural-selection defiance, and post-expiration-date opportunity, to mutate) won't let it pass?* So maybe your appropriately high level of leptin with your chronically full stomach does cross the blood-brain, but when it gets to the hypothalamus, the receptors that receive it don't quite "know" what to do with it? Or maybe the receptors do work, but one of the numerous downstream interdependent reactions fails?

There's another issue; it's social. If stroking a warm and fuzzy pet can lower your blood pressure, it would seem reasonable that the general environment in which your psyche functions should certainly carry the potential to affect hormones and thus, DNA expression.

Let me illustrate the point with a true cat story. Months ago, an unneutered longhaired gray feral cat paid a visit to the front yard of my home. The property has long been a lure for homeless creatures because it's walled off from the outside. While not encouraging these visitors, I usually can't resist and start feeding them. This gray longhaired cat was of normal weight with the usual pieces of missing ears from his testosterone-driven fights with other males. He wasn't particularly friendly, but wasn't particularly mean-spirited either. Soon, another unneutered black-and-white male feral cat of equal size, normal weight and the usual ear defects, appeared. Neither the gray nor black-and-white feral cats had anything to do with each other. They would occasionally posture from a distance, but never fought. They both eat and both filled out a bit, but remained slim for the next several months.

Enter a giant neutered tabby dropped off by someone who probably got tired of feeding him with hard-earned money in tight financial times. This giant neutered tabby was friendlier, but nevertheless aloof. The gray and black-and-white ferals stayed away from the newcomer and each other. Over the next few months, independently, the two unneutered ferals approached the neutered tabby with typical male-cat slow-motion movements and soft growls when the food dishes were freshly filled.

And then one day it happened while I watched. The gray feral finally got close enough to neutered tabby to receive a sudden closed-paw punch to his face with such force that it nearly knocked him over. Stunned, the gray feral just stood in place, demonstrating not even a hint of reactive aggressiveness nor panicky retreat. The neutered tabby looked away and stuck his face in the food dish.

Not long after, the black-and-white feral got into the act and received his own punch from the neutered tabby that I also witnessed. The black-and-white feral's response was nearly identical to the gray feral's.

Fast-forward a few months and the three cats are inseparable 24/7. They are now known as the three *amigos*. Every morning when I exit the front door, the threesome emerge from the bushes as one. A three-cat serenade of hunger follows. And then, the morning ritual of a closed-pawed punch to the faces of both unneutered feral cats, who take it not only as if expected, but seemingly with controlled gratefulness with the knowledge that their protector remains in good form. What's the point? These three cats, two originally of low weight and one of average weight are now fat as pot-bellied pigs! They constantly meow for food even when their dishes aren't empty.

Hypothesis: Two feral cats subjected to their natural environment competed for territorial dominance in order to procure enough nourishment for survival; they remained active in their search for sustenance and faced challenges from competitors that could endanger their lives; this stress was "appropriate" and genetically friendly even for a species whose DNA has been tainted by domestication; these two feral cats stumble into a nirvana; they remain vigilant and wild, trusting nothing but the food dish; they meet a suspected enemy whose initial lack of aggression is surprising; this prospective competitor asserts his dominance without violent battle; a new harmony provides food <u>and</u> protection with no effort and the naturally hostile world, with its "healthy" stresses and gene signaling, goes to hell in a hand basket; *leptin no longer works, and obesity reigns.* Sound familiar? Ask yourself, when was the last time you felt dangerously threatened when you approached the frozen-food section in a grocery store?

Recognizing that in the appropriate patient, bariatric surgery (see section: "WHAT'S THE DEAL WITH BARIATRIC SURGERY? *Evolutionary impatience*") has proven medically sound with significant improvement in morbidity and mortality, what else might we do aside from shopping for a larger pair of pants or dress?

First, address the problem and realize that you are at a biological disadvantage whether responsible or not. Use this reality for *motivation*, rather than moping over it. And understand that, leptin aside, if you try hard enough almost any otherwise healthy person can gain weight and that speaks for the opposite as well. And that many patients I have treated over the years, who are convinced that they, despite drastic calorie restriction and plenty of exercise, cannot lose weight, eventually do. I sometimes remind them that the First Law of Thermodynamics says that the 120-calorie piece of bread could not be responsible for ten additional pounds on their asses. It really is often a matter of incentive, such as that upcoming wedding or high school reunion or, unfortunately, the bad news from the doctor, which proves the point.

Tricks don't work. Quick fixes, often justified by patients as "jump starting," don't address the real issue, which is *long-term lifestyle change*. While rates of metabolism do vary from patient to patient, don't mislead yourself into the common practice of "wishful-thinking" calorie counting; patients, more often than not, underestimate calories by inaccurately estimating portion size.

The *source of your calories* probably does matter. While it's hard to imagine that every calorie is not the same, genetic research has identified a subset of overweight individuals who seem to gain more weight with intake of carbohydrate-calories when compared to the same calorie intake from non-carbohydrate sources. That having been said, there's ample evidence linking excess intake of carbohydrates in general with obesity and an associated tendency to diabetes.

Another issue might be mentioned here. Perhaps surprising to some, *sleep deprivation* can be a potential problem in that it *suppresses leptin*; the last thing you need in your quest to lose weight is a *LOWER* level of the stuff that's supposed to suppress your appetite when it ain't working well in the first place. Furthermore, *sleep deprivation increases ghrelin*! My guess on this one is that your DNA recognizes sleeplessness as a sign of *nocturnal predator risk*, which means you better have really good energy stores, because you may need to run long and hard as hell to avoid being a midnight snack.

Perhaps second only to the partial and half-truths proposed ad nauseam by mass media relating to the advantages of vitamin supplements (see section: "VITAMINS . . . TOO MUCH OF A GOOD THING? *Voodoo vitamins and other deceptions*"), weight-loss entrepreneurs have recognized the vast market and plan tapping into it. While I accept that many of the organized programs are well-founded in science and can be successful, the selection for presentation of their exceptional results (be they average citizen or celebrity) sets a tone for the viewer that, while not necessarily disingenuous, promises more than it usually delivers and, more importantly, shifts the emphasis away from long-term personal responsibility, providing that overly optimistic breath of relief: <u>they</u> can help me.

Let's look at obesity realistically. Other than the obvious – restrict calories, eat fewer carbohydrates, and exercise more – what is this epidemic all about? *Evolutionarily, food and its processing is primarily related to survival. When your hungry pet devours its food and appears content, it has satisfied a biological need rather than voiced approval of the chef. Our evolved brain has expanded basic hormonal biological satisfaction into the realm of human pleasure. And with this fine-tuning of a trait designed primarily for the continuation of the species, there is payment due. Carbohydrates, when available in nature, were intended as a quick source of life-sustaining energy, not a challenge to manipulate into luxurious self-indulgence.*

So, here's what I'm saying. Own up to it: through no real fault of our own, our extended life, with its mutated DNA, has rewritten the rulebook of the natural world. We can't do anything about that. But the realization of this fact can, and should, act as a stimulus to recognize that a solution to the problem remains biologically feasible. If we can only understand the importance of weight loss and make an investment that [despite what may seem high upfront costs (a bit of "inconvenience" and hunger)], will guarantee returns far more valuable than what Wall Street might ever offer, we can succeed. And at the same time, thumb our noses at MN.

IS LOWER BLOOD PRESSURE ALWAYS BETTER?

Going beyond therapeutic?

Most people know that "high blood pressure" is not a good thing. My guess is that fewer people know that low blood pressure can also not be a good thing. I suspect that neither group really understands what blood pressure really is. So, to the blackboard.

The left side of our heart (the *left ventricle*) receives oxygenated blood from our *lungs* (the "rejuvenated," red-in-color blood having first collected in a heart chamber called the *left atrium*). The *left ventricle* is the thickest of all four heart chambers and is responsible for generating enough pressure to push open an important one-way check valve (the *aortic valve*) between itself and the main blood vessel coming out of the top of the heart (the *aorta*). The pressure generated by the *left ventricle* must propel blood to every blood vessel in our bodies from head to toe, bringing circulation to our skin and other surface organs as well as to all our internal organs.

So then, the "top" number of your recorded blood pressure is the maximal pressure generated as the *left ventricle* squeezes down (so-called *systolic blood pressure*). The "bottom" number (the so-called *diastolic blood pressure*) is the remaining pressure in our arteries in-between heartbeats when the left ventricle relaxes. So, that famous 120/80 is the pressure in millimeters of mercury (each unit of pressure generated by a column of mercury, one millimeter tall), at its highest and lowest measurement during cardiac cycles. Without our aortic check valve, our pressure would read 120 over zero, because all the blood in our aorta would have rushed back into our left ventricle. This aortic-check-valve apparatus is important, at least in part, because the openings to our *coronary arteries* (that supply blood to the heart muscle itself) branch off from our aorta just beyond the aortic valve and thus get most of their blood supply while the heart rests between beats.

Okay, we've got the very basic anatomy of the left side of the heart [the *right side* is a different issue (see below) and intimately related to systemic blood pressure, but more than we need to know for this section] and how it relates to those numbers we see on those machines in the pharmacy, or on the screens of a myriad of cute little devices people buy in diligent response to their physician's recommendation or, thank goodness less often, as an outlet for obsessive preoccupation with concern that a high number, even once, is likely to cause a stroke. For those patients on adequate therapy who present me with long written lists of variable blood pressure readings they've recorded from early morning to when they finally drift off to sleep at night, I explain that fluctuating blood pressure, within certain limits depending on the circumstances, is normal. The example I frequently cite is that of a trained super-healthy athlete.

Let's say that we have a 17-year-old teenager, a Mr. or Miss or Ms. Let's choose a guy and make him a high-school track star whose parents are both still alive and well at age 100. We'll call him "Joe Perfect." This kid is so damn healthy that university doctors want his DNA for longevity experiments. His resting blood pressure is 120/80. So, one day a university doctor gets Joe to agree to let him install a painless pin-head-sized device under Joe's skin that measures his blood pressure continuously by beaming it up to a satellite. Now let's follow Joe on the day of a big race.

Wakes naturally and stretches: 120/80; remembers it's big-race day: 130/80; eats a light breakfast (an English muffin) and has a big cup of black coffee: 135/85; relaxes by playing with his dog: 125/80; drives to school and nearly gets into an accident when someone runs a stop sign: 150/90; talks to his teammates in the locker room, who remind him how they are counting on him to win the 200 meter dash: 160/80; completes his warm-up, checks the program and sees that in the past he has easily beaten all the athletes in his first heat: 110/75; standing on the starting line: 160/80; runs the first half of the race: 180/85; crosses the finish line: 200/90; takes a victory lap: 150/80; sits with his grateful buddies waiting for a pizza: 118/75.

The obvious point is that variability in one's blood pressure is normal. Perhaps the less obvious point is that this variability in blood pressure (including very high numbers) is a gift from MN in that it bestows a major survival advantage. If Joe Perfect was actually an antelope grazing on the Serengeti Plain with a normal blood pressure for such a creature and a cheetah charged, its life would depend on a coordinated biological response that includes delivering lots of blood to its leg and pelvic muscles for a run that could be its last. In both human "Joes" and animal "Joes," the visual, or emotional, response to alarming or threatening circumstances *immediately* increases the secretion of certain hormones, including those from our *adrenal glands* that sit on top of each kidney (for example, *epinephrine*, more commonly known as *adrenaline*), which accelerate heart rate, induce greater force of heart contractions, raise blood pressure, open arteries supplying leg and pelvic muscles and shunt blood away from other momentarily less important bodily functions (not a great time to "waste" blood by assigning it to the job of digesting an English muffin or grass).

Alright, the next logical question is: "What then is pathologically high blood pressure, and why do humans get it when antelopes probably don't?" Well, to start with, it's that same old story: Any antelope with a significant genetic defect contrary to survival would probably be eliminated before it could reproduce. There are no bow-legged or one-eyed antelopes routinely outrunning predatory cats. In the case of humans our mutated brains provide an unfair advantage so we live longer than we're supposed to in defiance of MN's law of natural selection. This delay in dying plays into the hands of spontaneous mutations, which can be good or bad, but must be seen in the context of a hell of a lot of DNA that is passing from cell to cell despite exceeding its "best-used-before" label. And this reality of our "artificial" (from the viewpoint of the bulk of our DNA not directly related to our superior intelligence) extension of life is, in my opinion, probably responsible for nearly everything health-wise that goes wrong in our lives when we reach age fifty or sixty; and this includes pathologically high blood pressure. And, one must add to this, the cultural "opportunities" that longevity provides as we so eagerly pursue non-biologically essential endeavors such as fast food, refined sugar, flame-retardant furniture and carpets, the convenience of plastic food containers, and even that new-car smell of a treasure trove of chemicals.

With all this having been said as background, let's briefly go back to our "Joe Perfect" for a moment. When he bends down to re-tie the shoelaces on his spikes after his warm-up, something internal and unknown to him occurs: he pools about a half to one liter of blood in the veins in his legs and pelvis while he kneels. You see, blood returns to the *right side of his heart* from his lower extremities by a "milking" process in that every time a muscle contracts it pushes blood up towards the right side of his heart (which includes low-pressure chambers called the **right atrium** and the **right ventricle**) with the help of check valves located in our larger veins that permit the movement of venous blood in one direction only.

Laces tied, "Joe Perfect" suddenly stands. This trapped blood doesn't move at the speed of light, so, for a **brief moment**, the **right side of his heart** and then his lungs, and then the **left side of this heart**, have just a little less blood in them than when he was warming up, and this in turn means that the amount of blood being pumped through his aorta is also of lower volume and thus his blood pressure is a bit lower than when he was kneeling.

This lower blood pressure is detected in specialized tissue (the **carotid sinuses**) in the arteries in his neck (the **carotid arteries**). MN has assigned these carotid sinuses the critical task of making certain that the brain is **always** perfused with an adequate volume and pressure of oxygenated blood. The carotid sinus cells detect the drop in pressure and through impulses sent to specialized areas in the brain trigger adjustments in the body that include a clamping down of blood vessels in the lower extremities and an acceleration of heart rate, which in turn restores the blood pressure and the flow of blood to Joe's brain. Despite all that just happened, "Joe Perfect" is clueless. You see, in a healthy person all these remarkable adjustments happen so quickly, it's as if there never was a potential problem in the first place.

Okay, let's move on to patients with pathologically high blood pressure. First of all, untreated high blood pressure is, in fact, a killer. Smaller blood vessels never evolved in humans adequately to accommodate a pounding of their delicate walls over long periods of time. This is true of every blood vessel in our bodies, but the vessels feeding the heart, brain, gastrointestinal tract and the delicate vessels in the outer layer of our kidneys (**glomeruli**) that filter waste products from our blood are particularly vulnerable. Combine high blood pressure with any of the recognized risks for vascular disease (high LDL cholesterol, diabetes, smoking, obesity and family history, for example) and you compound the problem. So, pathologically high blood pressure demands treatment.

Growing up, my maternal grandfather had high blood pressure. As a young kid, (even then I had some interest in medicine), I recall my grandfather having problems with the medications prescribed. Today I recognize that back then, other than diuretics, there were only two other lousy options for treatment in an active man of normal weight. The physician's choices boiled down to: do you want your patient to stand up and pass out (common side effect of a medicine called *Aldomet*), or get depressed as hell (common side effect of a medicine called *Reserpine*)? Fortunately today, it's a whole new ballgame (see below). We have available a diverse palette of medications for blood pressure control, many of which provide additional benefits to patients (preservation of kidney function in diabetic patients, and control of certain abnormal heart rhythms to name only two).

I would estimate that nearly 80% of my older patient population requires therapy for high blood pressure. Almost all of them can be controlled with one or more medications. Great! Good job doc. So why the title of this section: "IS LOWER BLOOD PRESSURE ALWAYS BETTER? *Going beyond therapeutic?*")?

A hint comes with the recent changes in the recommendations for what should be considered elevated blood pressure requiring therapy in various age groups.

The proposal put forth by an expert panel and published in a prestigious journal adjusts the acceptable "normal" blood pressure upward. More specifically, one recommendation raises the target in patients age 60 and older, settling on a therapeutic goal below 150/90. While I respect the panels' work, the very idea of setting a specific number for a specific age group is like saying an entire patient population has one of several identical fingerprints! Every patient, irrespective of age, is unique with specific medical needs. I have patients in their late 80s whose "correct" or "normal" systolic blood pressure (defined as the number that maintains the patient in a state of vascular compensation with no adverse symptoms or effects on lifestyle and with no laboratory evidence of injurious effects on other organs such as the kidneys) is 95! And I have patients in the same age bracket who feel like hell if their systolic blood pressure drops below 160. But the point here is not to criticize the new recommendations, but rather to recognize the legitimate concern implied whenever you shoot for a specific number, particularly in patients over the age of 60. If you target 120/80 in the elderly, especially if polypharmacy (using more than one group of drugs) is required, there is a real danger of dropping their blood pressure enough to cause them to stumble or pass out (***syncope***) with the potential for devastating injuries such as fractured hips. There are many visits to emergency rooms and hospitalizations in this age group because they were inadvertently overmedicated.

As mentioned earlier, today, physicians can choose from a wide variety of very effective drugs to control high blood pressure. These drugs work through various mechanisms and sometimes do have to be combined for the desired result.

One family of drugs (***ACE inhibitors*** or ***angiotensin converting enzyme inhibitors***) blocks an enzyme that reduces the amount of a substance in the blood that constricts the muscle layer in the walls of blood vessels as seen in high blood pressure. A related family of drugs blocks the effect of the vasoconstrictor substance at the muscle wall itself (these are called ***ARBs*** or ***angiotensin receptor blockers***).

Another group of antihypertensive drugs blocks the entry of calcium into the muscle in the wall of constricted blood vessels (these agents are called ***calcium channel blockers*** or ***calcium channel antagonists***), resulting in a dilatation and the lowering of blood pressure.

Yet another group (the **beta receptor blockers** or **beta antagonists**) blocks (gum-up in a sense) receptor sites on the heart's natural pacemaker cells, the heart muscle itself (particularly, if over-stimulated in a pathological state) and on the muscle cells in blood vessels. Their biochemical consequence is attenuation of the effects of **adrenaline** (**epinephrine**), and thus they slow the heart, counter a detrimental over-stimulated state within heart muscle, and dilate constricted vessels. The main result for purposes of this discussion? Blood vessel diameter increases and blood pressure goes down.

Diuretics or "water pills" rid the body of excess salt and water and thus, by reducing blood volume, decrease blood pressure.

Other drugs work on other receptor sites, and some even work in the brain to cause blood vessels to relax.

Finally, to make the essential point of this section, let's go back to our friend "Joe Perfect," but with some changes. He looks the same on the outside after his warm up before the race. He bends down to re-tie the shoe laces on his spikes (just as he did earlier) and then we get down and dirty. Through the miracle of literary license, I age his internal organs by about fifty years and place therapeutic levels of all the blood pressure lowering medications I listed above in his system. Now, while he's kneeling and working on his laces, despite my mischief, his blood pressure remains nice and normal. Then, he stands up and the shit hits the fan. There's even more pooled blood in his legs than before because some of his medications dilate veins as well as arteries. Even less blood goes to the right side of his heart, and through his lungs, and to the left side of his heart and up to his carotid sinuses that get the message of really low blood pressure. His carotid sinuses dutifully sound the "alarm." The alarm travels through his nervous system to his brain a little slower in our amended Joe. When the brain finally gets the message it frantically calls on its entire orchestra to play pretissimo! So what happens? The blood vessels in his legs receive the urgent message to constrict like Joe's life depends on it, but they're asleep at the wheel (with all our meds on board it's more like the vessels are slow at the wheel). His brain barks the command to the heart to triple time and squeeze with the power of a python on steroids, but the medications won't permit it. So poor Joe, with his youthful exterior and Medicare-age interior swimming with FDA-approved medication lies there on the ground, gravity alone restoring significant blood flow to his confused brain as an indignant MN stands over him and shakes her head with disgust. "Next time play by my rules."

So remember, high blood pressure is a killer, but any treatment should never be worse than the disease. Along this line, you should realize that if you're a new patient in a physician's office or visiting an urgent care facility or emergency room (for any reason), your recorded blood pressure might be higher than your usual pressure under ordinary, less stressful, circumstances. A well-intentioned physician, who may not know you or your propensity to handle stress with outside calm and internal chaos, might prescribe an unnecessary blood-pressure lowering agent, the unintended result? A re-visit to the facility after you got up out of your neighbor's car and hit the pavement.

When appropriately prescribed, *take your medication or medications regularly. Watch for signs of lightheadedness or dizziness, especially with position change* (not to be confused with moving-your-head-from-side-to-side dizziness, which is often an inner ear problem (See section: "IS DIZZY DANGEROUS? *The balance of balance*"). *If you notice symptoms with position change have someone take your blood pressure both lying down and then standing. Irrespective of the recording, report to your care provider at least by phone, or, if it's after hours and you're uncomfortable, have someone drive you to the nearest health-care facility.* But don't be surprised if MN slashes your driver's tires.

ARE ANTIBIOTICS
ALWAYS THE ANSWER?

Play the game, take the blame–badass bugs

Fossil evidence suggests that around 3 billion years ago some form of single-cell life existed. Fast forward (very fast) and here we are–humans! If not ironic, then at least intriguing, our bodies, both inside and out, are colonized with trillions of single-cell organisms called *bacteria*. The DNA in these guys isn't surrounded by a special membrane (the package called the *nucleus*), but rather sort of swims freely within the cell in its liquid contents, called *cytoplasm*, which does have an outer membrane that is additionally wrapped in a *cell wall* made of *sugar derivatives* and *amino acids* and serves primarily as a protective envelope, allowing certain essential materials in and out.

Now let's focus on one important group of these microscopic curiosities. We often hear their name as just *Staph* (not to be confused with *staff*, the people running around your doctor's office cursing insurance companies). The more accurate designation for this particular clan of interest is *Staphylococcus aureus*

(Aureus is Latin for "golden—more later). About a third of individuals carry this particular bug. These bacteria can live all over our skin with a special affinity for the tropical breezes and humidity in our *noses*. They generally get along with us as decent neighbors, partially because our natural immunity (like a neighborhood watch) keeps them in line. But, if we suffer from a variety of illnesses, the relationship may change. So, for example, if we are diabetic, or on dialysis for kidney failure, or immunocompromised for any reason, the truce is broken and these little buggers can create some problems ranging from an annoying pimple on your face (just in time for the class reunion), to very serious illnesses such as infected bones (*osteomyelitis*), *pneumonia*, infected membranes surrounding the brain (*meningitis*), infected heart valves (*endocarditis*) or even an overwhelming infection in our blood (*sepsis*).

Because these bugs often spread by skin contact, infections, often minor at first, more commonly appear when large numbers of people congregate in close quarters. So, individuals frequenting day-care centers, prisons (no comparison between the two implied), nursing homes, and even locker rooms are more likely to notice a scratch or a bruise that gets infected with staph.

From MN's viewpoint, staph infections (hopefully fatal) are just punishments for an "unnatural" longevity. You can imagine how irate she must have been when one of these intellectual upstarts, named Alexander Fleming, in 1928, noticed that a mold (*Penicillium notatum*) knocked the hell out of a colony of staph. But it wasn't until 1939, when the potential clinical applications of the substance was realized, that efforts to produce *penicillin* in large quantities got off the ground.

Now, here we are years later and so much smarter that we have cell phones, and yet our landfills brim with non-biologically degradable junk. Where am I going with this? Let me begin with a brief true story. When I was a medical resident in Southern

California, I moonlit occasionally. The experiences I encountered were often unexpected (they didn't tell me I had to deliver babies), but frequently enlightening.

One night, I found myself working the emergency room at a tiny hospital in the boondocks. At the time, there was an epidemic of a minor, self-limiting viral upper respiratory illness whose worst symptom was a barely recognizable drop or two of clear fluid drizzling from a baby's nose.

Late that night, several babies were brought in to the ER by well-intentioned parents whose young ones looked, and no doubt felt a hell of a lot better than I did. I carefully examined the babies and concluded that each of them had a mild case of the virus that was about as virulent as a cup of chamomile tea. But no matter how carefully, how respectfully I explained my diagnosis and the excellent prognosis with *no* medical therapy, every one of the families insisted that I prescribe an antibiotic or else clearly I must be an imposter in a white coat. How I ultimately responded is another story and beside the point, which is that way too many viral illnesses (that don't respond to antibiotics) are routinely treated with prescribed antibiotics.

The over-prescribing of antibiotics is a worldwide problem with a long history. In many countries, anyone can walk into a pharmacy and take home a variety of antibiotics without a prescription. Animals for eventual slaughter are often treated with antibiotics with the intention of accelerating their growth. For now, the take-home message here is simply that human ingenuity has placed a lot of survival stress on bacteria in general.

Let's go back to our uninvited cohabitant, ***Staph aureus***. I need not bore you with the chemistry of penicillin and similar antibiotics except to explain that the molecules are arranged in a way that includes a "ringed" structure (***beta-lactam ring***) as part of their chemical configuration, which has been very effective in killing staph by preventing it from accomplishing a critical biochemical maneuver in the production of its *cell wall*. An M&M candy is just not an M&M without its shell.

So, for more than a decade, penicillin worked just fine against *Staph aureus*, until somebody around 1950 got suspicious when treating patients with *Staph aureus* infections in the hospital setting. Guess what? Only about 60% of the bugs were effectively eliminated. Something had happened to a significant number of these bacteria that granted them immunity to a previously universally effective drug.

By the late 1950s, human brainpower kicked in and the structure of penicillin was modified (but still contained the beta-lactam ring) and the new upgraded penicillin called *methicillin* was born.

But in 1961, guess what? A new strain of *Staph aureus* was discovered in the lab (not cultured from a patient) that *no longer responded to Methicillin*. This *Methicillin-Resistant Staphylococcus aureus* is thankfully labeled more simply as *MRSA*. Seven years later, a *human case* infected with the resistant staph was discovered. But this bug was still very sensitive to another antibiotic (*vancomycin*), whose structure does not include a beta-lactam ring, but nevertheless interferes with the making of the bacterial cell wall. Done with this scary cat-and-mouse game? Not quite (and after the next few paragraphs you'll understand why the game may never end).

In 2002, the first *vancomycin-resistant staph* bug was discovered. Since then, this resistant organism is cropping up in increasing frequency in a variety of venues.

So what's going on here with this super bug? This little potential pest (or worse) may be small in size, but it's big in accumulated evolutionary advantage. After all, its earliest ancestors (*penicillin-sensitive Staph aureus*) have probably been around a lot longer than we have. While unprovable, some dinosaurs may have been covered from head to toe with it. But whatever its history, that predated humans, we were the ones who, at least in the first round of our science, knocked it on its metaphoric ass by the magic drug called penicillin. What I'm really saying is that <u>*we, with our overuse of drugs like penicillin, are responsible, in large part, for muscling a disproportionate (in an evolutionary sense) survival challenge on an organism that reproduces so quickly and is privy to mechanisms that can potentially condense eons of human evolution into days or less*</u>. I can see MN, in proud defense of her microscopic children who play by her rules, admonishing us: "You played the game, now take the blame."

And here's how the little bastards did it. Let's say that out of many billions of **Staph aureus** bacteria at the turn of the century (constantly subjected to random mutations, and dutifully exterminated by penicillin), one lucky guy hit the genetic jackpot and wound up producing a protein that just happened to split open the chemical ring that made penicillin effective in killing its brothers and sisters. In the staph community this is one very special celebrity with a unique talent. At risk for the stunted legacy resembling "one hit wonder," MN, in defense of bacterial innocence, has provided them with more than the usual method of passing on one's gift to one's offspring. Called **binary fission**, bacteria can double their DNA and split into two identical copies of themselves.

MN's evolutionary goodies include a "trick" called **horizontal transfer**, which allows our celebrity bacterium to pass its anti-penicillin gene directly to a neighbor. So, down the road, we've got lots of staph that thumb their metaphoric noses at Dr. Fleming's great discovery, but are still destroyed by one of the updated penicillin-like drugs such as **methicillin**. Guess what? Billions of penicillin-resistant, methicillin-sensitive staph are exposed again and again to methicillin and (you probably guessed it), one bug is blessed with a mutation in a gene that now codes for a protein that just happens to nullify the killing effects of methicillin and so **MRSA** is born. This so-called **mecA gene** can also be passed on to other bacterial cells in a number of ways, which disseminates this newly developed weapon against humanity. And it doesn't stop here. As mentioned earlier, antibiotics that were routinely effective against MRSA (such as *vancomycin*) are coming up short in certain cultures taken from infected patients. *It's always been a race between what we as an intelligent species can manufacture in the lab and our competition, which has passively evolved through mutation and responded to the survival stress we have placed upon it. And in that process, we have predisposed bad bugs to develop into "badder" bugs.*

Aside from antibiotic resistance, **Staph aureus,** in step with MN's "survival of the fittest" mantra, has loaded itself with nasty products to help perpetuate itself at the expense of its host. Some examples: the yellow color of the bug (remember what aureus means in Latin?) is a pigment *(staphyloxanthin)* that interferes with our immune systems ability to kill it; it makes enzymes *(hyaluronidases)* that attack the integrity of our cells, basically softening them up so it can spread more easily; it makes a protein that causes our plasma to clot (this so-called **coagulase** makes it tougher to get our immune response to the site of infection); and it makes a variety of other toxic substances that help dissolve any host cellular component that gets in its way. And much of this devilishness is packaged in units floating around in the staph cell, sometimes brought there with the help of viruses (**bacteriophages**), which create another method for passing on "bad-for-people" genes to neighboring bacterial cells.

Now that you have decided to abandon your home for life in a sterile bubble, a little bit of good news. Overall, the rate of serious **Staph aureus** infections is down. Since the bug is most often spread by hand contact with contaminated surfaces (for example, doorknobs, keyboards and bed sheets), the recent emphasis on providing easily accessible dispensers of antiseptic soaps and washes (even grocery stores have them) has helped. (This "protective" methodology has recently generated some long-term concerns). But irrespective of all mentioned in this paragraph, remember there are a significant number of carriers out there whose nasal membranes are colonized with MRSA; so an uncovered sneeze can infect a vulnerable person. Also, remember that disrupting the integrity of your skin, whether it is from scratching an itch or following the insertion of an IV line, careful follow-up is required. ***Redness, pain, swelling, the obvious collection of awful looking material (I hate the "P" word) at the site of trauma should sound the alarm.***

We've come a long way on this subject of importance. The lesson here goes beyond the obvious; the game we play, using our brains to coexist (MN might prefer the word *subvert* rather than *co-exist*) with nature, carries a real risk. Our interventions are understandably self-serving, but immediate gratification can blind one from seeing the future. Some would challenge our species' status as recent arrivals, preferring the designation of uninvited guest.

And in all this stunning, miniscule reality we have reviewed in this section, there is an unexpected irony: left to evolution as MN sees it (spontaneous mutations subject to probabilities that are more likely than not to avoid revolutionary change, since radical alterations in physical or biochemical characteristics tend to confer survival disadvantage rather than advantage), neither we nor Staph aureus, at least in our current forms, should exist.

HOW DO I KEEP
MY BONES STRONG?

Aging ladies, watch your step

S ay the word *bone* and our brains conjure up the image of a
static, bleached skeleton of some long-dead creature under a
cactus in a desert. Living bone is the antithesis of that portrait.
The bone in us (antemortem status assumed since dead people
won't be reading this book) is a dynamic, constantly active tissue.
It repairs and eloquently responds to stress, toughening itself in accommodation. So what changes? What goes wrong when a woman
reaches menopause and after a bone density test is told her obsta-
cle course days must go the way of the bikini, and MN impatiently
and dispassionately waits for that fall and that fractured hip, thinking: "Finally–better late than never."

I'll focus on women in this section only because, as unfair as it
may appear, men fracture hips at a significantly lower rate than the
female of the species. This is probably, at least in part, the result of
a greater lifelong muscle mass in men, which stresses bone continuously and predisposes to higher density, and the dependency and

later withdrawal of estrogen (you'd think MN could identify) and the loss of its potent, positive effects on bone density in women. More later on this important subject.

But we're getting ahead of the story. If you think about it, it makes perfect sense that the bones of youth are plastic in function. How else could a bone heal? And if you've ever seen a chest x-ray of a 20-year-old body builder versus your 100-year-old aunt, who claims that her longevity is somehow related to the intellectual stimulation afforded her by sitting on her couch ten hours a day watching soaps and game shows, you would realize that healthy *stress* on young bones makes them denser and that little or *no stress* on older bones makes them less dense.

Think about the *disadvantage* to an established species if a per-fectly good set of genes, potentially replete with not-yet-evident survival advantages, was sacrificed from expression in a future generation because its own testosterone fooled it into thinking it was experienced and strong enough to win a physical battle with an older, more skillful male overseeing a harem of females. So, this "ego" inflated amateur with some decent DNA goes toe to toe with a Godzilla of the species and in defeat fractures a few ribs, or other bones, in his lost battle.

The vanquished limps off to lick his wounds and rethink a failed strategy. Now, our lover boy may still not survive if some-thing higher on the food chain immediately goes after his butt, but, if he's lucky, he'll have time to heal his injured bones and get another chance at love next year. You see, MN has apparently decided that bone injury forcing modest disability should not be a deal breaker when it comes to the passage of DNA. If it was to be a final event for the injured, there would be no mechanism for re-pair, and sooner or later our four-legged Casanova would bite the dust, his DNA lost. You might argue: So what if each injured chal-lenger died? Wouldn't the best beast for the job eventually come along, the gene pool of his species benefiting then? The counter to that is it's not just strength alone that empowers survival advantage; it's things like cunning, tenacity and ability to learn. It's likely that those traits, expressed genetically, contributed to the ascension of humans from lower primates?

So now let's look at how our living bodies, in a healthy and youthful state, respond to broken bones. Some understanding of this is important before we explore the critical topics of diminished bone density, proposed (often controversial) therapy, and the growing incidence of fractured hips with devastating impact on individuals, families and the health care system, all of which means diddly to MN as she laments over the survival of any women after menopause.

The physiology of the adaptive mechanism of bone healing is both complex and still not fully understood. While there are many cell types contributing their evolutionary "expertise" to the process, let's start with two of the main characters in and around bone.

One cell type is essentially a bone "eater" (*osteoclast*) and the other is essentially a bone "maker" (*osteoblast*). Let's put enough stress on one of your bones to create a tiny microscopic crack, nothing that would even trigger a visit to the emergency room.

Now let's go microscopic and see what happens. The mature bone cells (*osteocytes*) in the crack die (from the trauma). The mature bone cells nearby detect the crack and the death of their buddies and secrete substances that join the *"bone-surface" cells* more intimately with tiny *blood capillaries* (this allows certain "stuff" in the blood, such as other cells that will be needed later, to have more direct access to the job site) and, at the same time, the living buddies of the newly deceased mature bone cells stimulate *another type of cell* that just happened to be sitting around near the bone surface passing the time of day. These "lazy guy" cells are then suddenly employed and transform into a more active cell, not yet ready for full-time work. These formerly "lazy guy" cells' part-time work includes transforming baby bone "eater" cells (osteoclasts) that swim in the blood into mature bone "eating" cells (pool party over, get to work). The party ends abruptly as these now-mature bone "eaters" go to town and eat their way through the crack, hollowing out additional bone (think of it as a dentist who has to prepare the site around a cavity in a tooth before he can place a filling).

The job of hollowing out the area around the crack completed, these bone "eaters" (formerly swim-party guys) essentially die (that's evolutionary gratitude for a job well done). Now, these formally "lazy guy," formerly part-time workers make their transformation into full-time bone "makers" (*osteoblasts*), as they get right to work collecting and applying the raw materials, such as *calcium* and *phosphorus*, and re-form the missing bone, returning it to normal. The assignment finished, MN rewards the hard work by selecting some of the bone "makers" for transformation into either bone "eaters," or "bone-surface" cells, or (the bitch that she can be) just kills them.

Okay, now to *calcium*, one of the most important minerals that give bones their hardness. Let me warn you here. I will make every effort to take you by the hand through what follows, but it's not easily palatable. You see, in order for any living system to maintain itself, safeguards must be in place to promote an ongoing balance of the concentrations of biologically active substances in blood and other organs. This is particularly true in maintaining normal bone density and is complex enough that even today in 2015, the physiologists who love this stuff still aren't completely certain what the hell *magnesium* does in the picture that follows. So in keeping with my bargain to go easy on you, I won't discuss magnesium.

A legitimate question by you at this juncture is: "Why bother with this bone chemistry stuff at all?" The answer is that even if you fly over what follows, appreciating its intricacy has value in your understanding of both how marvelous the machinery is and, perhaps more to the reason you bought this book in the first place, the differing medical opinions as to the best therapies for low bone density in women.

Back to <u>calcium</u>. As mentioned earlier, the concentration of any biologically active substance must be kept in balance; what goes in (for example, in one's diet) must be coordinated with what is used, or metabolically converted (essentially what goes out). If not? Fugetaboutit! Non-living things do just fine without this biological "complexity." While your aunt's antique table might last for a few centuries or longer, it can't repair a scratch by itself and it certainly isn't going to grow over time and eventually make little baby tables.

In the case of calcium, the essential balancing, or feedback, substance is a hormone called **parathormone**, abbreviated as **PTH** (this hormone is secreted by small glands imbedded in our **thyroid** called **parathyroid glands**), which **raises** our blood levels of calcium and drops the blood level of **phosphate** (more later).

A less-important player is a hormone called **calcitonin**, made by special cells in our thyroid, which **lowers** our blood calcium.

But it's not that simple. Enter **vitamin D**, which promotes bone resorption and **increases** calcium uptake from the gut resulting in a **rise** in blood calcium and also a **rise** in **phosphate**. Phosphate then counters vitamin D by inhibiting calcium absorption from the intestine, encouraging a ***drop*** in serum calcium. *The point is that, even at this very simplified level, you can see the elaborate nature of calcium metabolism and can better understand why, after years of research, there remains controversy over which supplements, and at what dose, are most beneficial as therapy for low bone density **(osteopenia).*** Remember, our DNA is the conductor of this symphony of biological activity, and while we understand one gene results in the production of one protein, the majority of our DNA has escaped our ability to figure out exactly what the hell it does.

So here you are, a female member of a species programmed to make children and then disappear, but also the benefactor of unprecedented intelligence that extends your survival, and just when you're old enough to enjoy the fruits of a lifetime of work and/or child rearing, your ovaries yawn and a lousy bone density test says "watch your step," literally. So, you've got to wonder, with a hint of optimism, what you or medical science might do to tap into all that mysterious DNA with unknown function and pull out of it some crumb of new knowledge that will allow you to sustain your femininity, put on your dancing shoes and boogie a bit longer with intact hips.

It's time to address *estrogen*, that hormone whose name is unquestionably synonymous with womanhood, but whose function, in all but the healthy youthful female, has driven researchers and clinicians absolutely nuts with decades of conflicting and confusing research results. What does it do to a woman's bone density (and her blood vessels) in addition to driving young men into obsession?

Simplifying something very complex, normal amounts of *estrogen* have two major effects on bone. Remember our bone "maker" cells? Well, these guys are stimulated to do their thing, which means *higher bone density.* And remember our bone "eater" cells? Well, estrogen basically shuts them down, resulting in *less bone resorption.* Nice combo, right? A hormone that does everything right if you're looking for bones of steel. So, what's the issue? Keep estrogen levels up as they naturally decrease in aging women and all is rosy, except in the orthopedic surgeon's office where he starts laying off staff. Well, for years doctors thought using estrogen replacement was a done deal: keep older women looking and feeling like their younger counterparts, nice skin, maintain that sharp intuition, keep coronary arteries clean, everything good. Then reasonably designed studies involving lots of women were performed and the brakes were applied.

In 1998, a study (known as the *HERS study*) recruited thousands of post-menopausal women (uterus intact) with known

vascular disease. The purpose of the study, lasting just over four years, was to determine if these women (already diagnosed with vascular disease) might benefit (slow the disease down) by treating them with a ***combination*** of ***estrogen*** and another female hormone called ***progesterone.*** Equal numbers of woman received sugar pills as a control (this was a double "blind" study because neither the docs nor the patients know who got what). The expectation was that these "youth" hormones should help, especially since vascular disease was a known affliction of older women. But guess what? The women taking the hormones had ***no reduction in adverse cardiac events*** and an ***increase in blood clots in the lungs***! The proposed possible silver lining extracted from this by the authors was their suggestion that one could argue that since cardiac events ***did not increase*** maybe these women (whose cardiac problems would have been expected to deteriorate over time) should, after all, be placed on the combination of hormones.

In 2002, another large-scale double-blind study (part of what is called the ***Woman's Health Initiative or WHI***) was conducted to better assess the possibility that estrogen and progesterone in combo might be helpful in ***preventing*** vascular disease in postmenopausal woman with ***no history or findings of vascular disease.*** Well, the trial was stopped early because there were serious problems developing in one of the groups (researchers call these groups "arms"). Turns out, the combination of hormones were demonstrating an ***increase in invasive cancer of the breast***, and an ***increase in adverse cardiovascular events, strokes and blood clots in the lungs.*** And once again there was a tarnished silver lining (apropos to our discussion) in that there was a ***significant reduction in hip fractures*** in the treated group. So, estrogen (at least in combination with another female hormone – progesterone) seems in the real world, and, as expected, benefits hip density and reduces hip fractures, but at an obviously extreme high cost, at least in the age group tested.

Now let's jump forward after years of additional studies that raked estrogen in combination progesterone over the coals. It seems logical to test whether estrogen alone qualifies as a "good witch" or a "bad witch" in the real world women with low bone density.

In 2012, the **U.S. Preventive Services Task Force**, a group of independent experts were asked by the government to investigate and summarize all the data collected since 2002, which included 51 studies evaluating both the combination of estrogen and progesterone and the use of estrogen alone. ***When the whole collection of studies was reviewed, the panel's recommendation was cautious, bordering on steadfast: Even in the estrogen alone group, the risks of long-term therapy appeared significant.***

Then, in 2013, a sophisticated statistical analysis performed by a group at Yale compared hysterectomized women, ages 50 to 59, in the general public (factoring in the decline of estrogen use based upon the studies and recommendations stated in the previous paragraph) to those who had received estrogen in those same studies, and arrived at a ***shocking conclusion: of those hysterectomized women, age 50 to 59, who stopped taking estrogen in response to the perceived risks of the hormone, there were approximately 50, 000 unnecessary deaths! The take home here (over and above the possible associations of heart disease, cancer, blood clots and mortality with estrogen therapy for improved bone density), as I suggested early on in this section, is that arriving at a recommendation is painfully complicated, in large part because the biology is not only beautifully elegant, but intertwined in still-secret sophistication that even our proposed intelligence has yet to penetrate.*** This reality of our persistent ignorance is further emphasized by the fact that, maybe surprisingly, estrogen alone reduces LDL ("bad" cholesterol), raises HDL ("good" cholesterol) in blood, which would be consistent with the conclusion reached in the 2013, statistical analysis just cited. Despite MN's grin, I will still make recommendations regarding the use of estrogen to improve bone density later in this section, admittedly based on a substantial degree of intuition as well as science.

So, what does a woman do in the practical world to maximize bone density and prevent hip fracture in later life? First look at the biology (I'll assume you hadn't fallen asleep, although I couldn't blame you). There is no question that weight bearing on bones increases their density. Those bone "maker" cells get busy and those bone "eater" cells take a nap. *It just makes sense; evolution and natural selection are smart enough to know that they must reward the agile and punish the lazy.* So, if you are female (especially female, but male as well), your DNA expects *regular exercise*. Disappoint it and pay the consequences as junk genes and detrimental stretches of DNA that don't code for known, "good" proteins turn on. *My specific recommendation is to engage in a combination of muscle strengthening and cardiac conditioning, starting at the first signs of the disappearance of one's baby fat.*

So, if you're a parent or grandparent advise your daughters and granddaughters to start early and make exercise part of their lives. And that means forever. If feasible, this also applies to you (especially if post-menopausal). Don't go overboard with the weights (resistance bands are even better and less likely to cause injury). I suggest lots of repetitions, upper and lower body, with light resistance. Avoid the temptation to keep increasing the load. Fifteen minutes a day is more than adequate.

For younger women, the cardio can be jogging (best for weight bearing), or brisk walking, or treadmill, or elliptical (less weight bearing), the last two especially helpful in motivating you if bad weather or minor aches and pains discourage you from brisk walking. A combination approach for the reasonably fit that saves time is twenty minutes of power walking with light (one to two pound) hand or wrist weights. Use no higher than two pounds of weight in each hand or on each wrist as a maximum, no matter how warrior-like you think you've become. Remember, for best results march with weighted arms pumping like you're on a military drill. This type of exercise is natural; we assume a posture that distributes our weight as our skeletal structure intended.

Okay, I see the sneers. "Great doc. On my next go round with life, I'll keep your suggestions in mind." *If you are unable to walk (march) with light weights (many menopausal woman in my practice, even in their eighties, still can) because of a disability, other than lack of motivation, a home treadmill with railings for support might still work. If that's not to your liking, or is still too difficult, gardening, or any household or recreational activity that uses major muscle groups and puts at least some conservative stress on your bones can be helpful. I've even told reluctant patients to use soup cans (unopened at my request because of their high-sodium content) as weights, extending their arms outward from their sides while standing (or even sitting) or lifting them over their heads.* Look, even that's better than nothing.

Let's move on to *calcium supplements* before and after menopause. Remember it is inappropriate to make the leap that a substance that is necessary for health automatically is healthier in higher amounts. This misconception forms the basis for shrewd marketing that keeps companies selling supplements in business.

The best way to handle calcium is dietary. Yes, you do need some milk products in your diet, despite what some might lead you to believe. But if you plan taking a calcium supplement, so long as your stomach makes acid, either *calcium carbonate* or *calcium citrate* will do. Remembering that no matter how much calcium you dump into your system, you have no guarantee (not even a rational wish) that all that stuff is somehow going to turn on your *osteoblasts* (bone "makers") and shut down you're *osteoclasts* (bone "eaters"). If you have low bone density *(osteopenia)* or full-blown *oseteoporosis*, there's a hell of a lot more going on biochemically in you than too little calcium. Taking into account the high biological probability that too much calcium is not a good thing, I recommend *no more than 500 to 750mg of calcium as a maximum per day.*

Vitamin D is a hot item. And when you're done reading the next paragraph that may be how your collar feels. Remember, vitamin D's primary function is to *raise serum calcium and phosphate levels* by increasing calcium absorption from your gut, and decreasing phosphate loss through your kidneys. The source from which vitamin D gets the calcium it uses to raise our blood levels is primarily *bone. Vitamin D deficiency reduces* calcium absorption from the gut, which lowers blood levels of calcium and this in turn provokes a countermeasure in the form of more *PTH* from our parathyroid glands, which helps correct the deficit by pulling more calcium from our bones and also, as another countermeasure, decreasing the loss of calcium through our kidneys. This "holding on" to calcium by the kidney promotes the loss of phosphate in the urine, because if equal amounts of calcium, and phosphate were absorbed in the kidney they would essentially "react" with each other, their formed complex removing them from doing anything "helpful" in our blood or bones.

Since bone is mainly calcium and phosphorus (the calcium and phosphate substance that makes bone hard is called *hydroxy-apatite*), this phosphate that is lost in the urine is basically pulled from the bones weakening them further. So you see, truly low levels of vitamin D trigger mechanisms to sustain blood levels of calcium (that's PTH's job that it dutifully performs) at the expense of bone density.

In severe cases of vitamin D (and usually calcium) deficiency present in extremely malnourished children, a condition called *rickets* can develop. You might Google rickets and see how severely the soft bones of legs deform with weight bearing. This is quite different from the low density, brittle bones seen in osteopenia or osteoporosis, but illustrates the point that every element biologically active in normal bone metabolism is essential.

Let's get practical with vitamin D. Since blood screening reveals that many Americans of all ages have deficient blood levels, the euphoria of "cure everything" with mega doses has caught on. Remember, a vitamin is a substance needed by the body in small quantities. While we get some vitamin D from our diets (fish oils and milk products, and sometimes through food additives), most of it is synthesized in our skin by sun exposure. But, in conflict with what MN intended for the young of the species, the computer age has substituted screen watching for outdoor playing. This coupled with legitimate concerns about sun-induced skin cancer; it's not surprising that researchers find low blood levels of vitamin D. But, there is controversy in the medical literature regarding what really constitutes a normal level. Remember ***vitamin D promotes bone resorption and increases calcium absorption*** from the gut to raise serum calcium levels. And its biological effects are coordinated with other minerals and hormones (as we so laboriously learned earlier). Do you really want to mess with that complexity by downing a ton of this vitamin because a label prepared by a marketing team with expertise in selling dish detergents claims it's "good for bone health?" If you answered *yes,* there's a witch doctor who claims a powdered root fertilized by the droppings of a mystical capybara is equally effective. Don't be fooled.

So looking over a bunch of stuff in the literature, it seems that blood levels of vitamin D (determined by the ***25-hydroxy vitamin D test***) are best kept somewhere ***between 20 to 50 ng/mL***. This is lower than some authors recommend, but seems to me both sensible and unlikely to cause problems. ***For people with limited sun exposure, appropriate blood levels can be probably achieved with 600 IU daily for teens through age 70; older people make and absorb less vitamin D so they may require 700 to 800 IU daily.***

Remember ***calcitonin?*** That's the hormone made by specialized cells in the thyroid and while not a major player in the complex mosaic of calcium metabolism, it does lower serum levels by inhibiting our bone "eating" cells and probably stimulating our bone "making" cells. ***One of its potential problems is that it significantly*** *increases calcium excretion in urine. If used over long periods of time, there may be significant risk to kidney function.*

Calcitonin is available as a nasal spray or an injection. It's actually a synthetic version of *salmon calcitonin*, which has similar effects as the human form, but is more potent (brand names are *Fortical* and *Miacalcin*). It should only be considered if other options are less suitable to an individual patient's medical needs, and they are at *least five years post-menopausal with osteoporosis and increased risk of fracture.* Furthermore, most of the data on calcitonin is relevant to fractures of the spine (*vertebral column*, or back bone) so its application for the prevention of hip fractures is not established. One potential niche for short-term therapy is that it seems to be fairly effective in reducing severe pain immediately following a fracture of the spine. As with most therapies for osteoporosis, adequate intake of calcium and vitamin D is essential if this intervention is to have even a prayer of working.

The most commonly prescribed drugs for osteoporosis with the hope of reducing the risk for a first-time, or subsequent, hip fracture are called the *bisphosphonates*. There are a lot of them out there for many reasons, including marketing opportunities generated by the growing number of aging baby boomers of the female gender. Some brand names you may recognize from either the bottle in your medicine cabinet or TV commercials include: *Didronel*, *Fosamax*, *Boniva*, *Actonel* and *Aclasta*. It's not entirely clear whether these drugs partially work through stimulating bone "making" cells (remember they're called *osteoblasts*), or (the more likely effect) by inhibiting (actually annihilating) bone "eating" cells (remember they're called *osteoclasts*).

These bone "eating" cell killer medications are poorly absorbed in the GI tract (an enteric coated version is available as well as an intravenous form), and can irritate the *esophagus*. That's why the pill form must be taken first thing in the morning on an empty stomach with lots of water and the requirement of sitting or standing for at least 30 minutes to an hour (depending on the product) to avoid the pill coming back up and into contact with the esophagus.

When these *bisphosphonates* finally reach bone, they stay there for a *very long time* (actually for years!). This is why the duration of therapy, from my vantage point, is a challenge and some physiologically oriented experts limit their use to no more than five years. It also concerns me, and others, that screwing around with the complexities of bone metabolism for an extended period of time is looking for trouble, this, despite the research that confirms that these medications do (perhaps not as impressively as many, including me, might hope) work. This potential problem is reflected in the well-reported, rare, but "unusual" kinds of fractures seen in patients using these medications. These include fractures in the *shaft* of the *femur* (leg bone from hip to knee) rather than the more common location (in the region of the neck of the femur where it joins to the side of the pelvis) as well as fractures in post-menopausal women's *jaws* with no recent history of professional boxing. All considered, my suspicion is that there are probably additional long-term adverse effects, especially if prescribed for younger women with only modest risk for hip fracture.

Since the mechanism of bone fracture and repair involves an intricate rebuilding of bone, and the "natural" interaction of our *osteoblasts* and *osteocyte*s during that stressed time must be in high gear, it raises the question whether it's smart to mess with nature at such a dynamic time with a bisphosphonate? This question, to date, has not been fully answered. But think about it. Here you are with DNA that says you're lucky as hell to be alive at a time when you can get a senior discount at a movie theater; your hormones, or lack thereof, are in the land of Oz far from your biological Kansas; you fracture your hip (the bitch MN nodding dispassionate approval) when you lift your two-pound Pomeranian; your beloved male doctor visits you in the hospital (he could trip over his medical bag a dozen times without fracturing anything other than his ego); your doctor gasps when he sees your bone X-ray, more for your lousy bone density than the tiny fracture, and proceeds to discuss the option of starting a medication that stays in your bones for more months than there are pages in *War and Peace*. Personally, I might wait until the fracture heals a bit.

Before discussing estrogen let's briefly talk about a related substance–drugs in the class that are called *Selective Estrogen Receptor Modulators* or *SERMS*. Their development was an attempt to find a molecule that would retain the benefits of estrogen on bone density in post-menopausal woman and minimize the potential adverse effects of the native hormone. The specific agent relative to this section is called *raloxifene* or *Evista*. While it does have positive effects in promoting higher bone density (but probably less so than bisphosphonates and "real" estrogen) and does have positive effects on cholesterol levels (like estrogen itself), and even blocks estrogen's effect on breast tissue, resulting in anti-breast-cancer benefits, it retains warnings that include a higher incidence of blood clots in veins, which may break off and get filtered out in lungs (a serious, potentially life-threatening condition called *pulmonary emboli*), and in post-menopausal women with *known coronary disease* is associated with an increased risk for *stroke* or *major coronary events*, this despite improving blood cholesterol (go figure).

Now, finally, to *estrogen* and its potential use in post-menopausal women with decreased bone density. Before I go any further, <u>*let me strongly emphasize that any possible use of estrogen in this setting should be discussed with a gynecologist or an endocrinologist. My recommendations are based on my reading of a complicated, not uncommonly conflicting, literature and intuition accumulated over time with an emphasis on "do thy patient no harm" and never waste an opportunity to fool MN.*</u>

There is no question that *estrogen* is highly effective in maintaining bone density over many years. Studies have proven that this fact *does* translate into reduced hip fractures. When examining the problems with this therapy, one should separate the studies that combined estrogen with progesterone from those that used estrogen alone.

In women, older than 60, who took *estrogen alone*, there was *no* increase in observed heart attacks, nor was there an increase in breast cancer, but there seemed some additional risk for strokes. In younger woman (under 60), the stroke risk *wasn't* evident. So, when we combine this with the beneficial effects of estrogen, and the statistical study that suggested withholding estrogen out of fear of its adverse effects in woman between age 50 and 59, may have resulted in high numbers of unnecessary cardiac deaths, it seems reasonable to consider <u>*solo estrogen therapy in this 50 to 59 year-old age group at significant risk for hip fracture. And then, after age 60, to consider an alternative therapy less likely to increase the risk of breast cancer, which increases with both natural aging and long-term exposure to supplemental estrogen*</u>.

Let's summarize this exhausting section. First of all, *try and avoid all the medical speculation/confusion by beginning and sustaining a life-style that incorporates appropriate weight-bearing exercise from at least the time of your first menstrual cycle to well beyond your last. Incorporate this bone-friendly activity into your life* with the same consistency as brushing your teeth or combing your hair. Remember, your DNA expects nothing less or (from an orthopedic standpoint) your bone density is most likely toast. *The more exercise you perform, the more likely you are to stymie MN into blinking with confusion as to how old you really are, no matter what your DNA says.* Now, if you're in the rapidly expanding group of women who remember running to the record shop for that first Elvis hit, and now the only running in your life requires nose drops, pass the message on to those younger ones whom you love.

Exercise a given (no matter what form it takes), you must remember that no medication will work unless you **supply enough raw material** to the job site. As outlined above, calcium and vitamin D are essential in physiologically appropriate amounts. Larger intakes of supplements will either do nothing or interfere with your goal or, worse yet, introduce some unrelated medical problem. Don't forget, we are one hell of a complicated organism with an extraordinary set of checks and balances that don't need any functional help from unregulated vitamin companies with big advertising budgets.

WHAT'S THAT FLUTTER
IN MY CHEST?

Atrial fibrillation–a valentine from Mother Nature

Way back when you were no more than a cluster of cells, the one-month product of a fertilized egg, and MN watched with all the love, enthusiasm and expectation of a first-time parent at a child's recital, a microscopic tube that would become your *heart* started contracting spontaneously. The first of your organs to demonstrate function, your heart forms by a series of miraculous maneuvers as cells line up, propagate, dance into positions, grow into sheets that descend and twist into a four-chambered structure that both biologically and poetically is the essence of our humanity.

The human heart has four chambers and looks very little like what appears on a Hallmark card. We divide the heart into the right and left side for good reason. The ***right side***, which includes an upper chamber (called the ***right atrium***) and a lower chamber (called the ***right ventricle***), is a low-pressure system. If we stuck a needle in either right-sided chamber, the blood would more drip than shoot out across the room. The reason for this low pressure is the right side of the heart, which contains blood from which our organs have removed much of the oxygen (dark and bluish in appearance and called *venous blood*) is pumped to our *lungs* (through a large blood vessel originating from our right ventricle and called the *pulmonary artery*), which are made up of delicate blood vessels and air carrying tubes (*bronchioles*) serving the purpose of allowing the carbon dioxide in our blood to leave (as we exhale) and oxygen from the air to enter as we breath in or inhale. Microscopic units, where the gases are actually exchanged (called *alveoli*), number around 300 million and provide a usable surface area often estimated as the size of a tennis court. So, you can understand that a high pressure entering so delicate a system would be like using a firehouse to inflate a tiny balloon.

Once our blood has been oxygenated in our lungs, it returns to the left side of the heart, which is also made up of two chambers. The upper chamber, which first receives the newly vitalized blood from our lungs (now redder in color with the addition of oxygen to a special protein called *hemoglobin* carried by our *red blood cells* or *erythrocytes*), is called the *left atrium*. This upper chamber on the left side of our heart pumps the blood into the lower, left-side chamber called the *left ventricle*. This left ventricle is thicker than its counterpart on the right side of the heart and generates a high pressure with its contractions. The blood exits the left ventricle through a big (the biggest) artery called the *aorta*. This higher pressure generated by the left ventricle is necessary because this rich, red oxygenated blood must reach every organ, every cell, in our body from our scalp to every internal organ to the bottoms of our feet, and that job doesn't get done with some wimpy force.

Okay, basic anatomy class dismissed. But wait a minute. Stop to think about it. Why doesn't the blood just slosh around in our hearts like a washing machine on its wash cycle? To begin with, our hearts have *four one-way check valves*, one between the right atrium and the right ventricle (called the ***tricuspid valve***), and one between the left atrium and the left ventricle (called the ***mitral valve***). There are also two additional one-way check valves, one at the exit of the right ventricle (on the way to the lungs) called the ***pulmonary valve***, and another valve at the exit of the left ventricle (on the way to our entire body) called the ***aortic valve***.

All right, four one-way check valves that keep our blood moving in one direction only. Problem solved? Not exactly. Back to our washing machine analogy. You've got to plug the damn thing into an electrical outlet or nothing happens.

Returning to the opening sentence of this section, at four weeks after conception heart cells (***myocytes***) start contracting. That means they have moved chemical substances (***ions***) in and out and across the biological envelopes that hold their contents (***cellular membranes***) in a fashion that generates an electrical impulse. Now think about it. If every heart cell in a mature four-chambered heart fired at the same time, we would have the *Guinness Book of World Records* biological fiasco with a cramp to end all cramps, and one very dead human. So, what's the deal here? In order for our four-chambered miracle to work, there must be a "brilliantly" coordinated series of electrical events and consequent contractions. Enter the ***conducting system*** of the human heart.

Near the top of our right atrium, the ***cardiac pacemaker*** (called the ***sinoatrial node***) sits. This remarkable tissue is constantly in electrical flux, spontaneously charging itself to deliver an impulse into the top chamber (***right atrium***) of our heart. This natural pacemaker is in close contact with our brain and circulating hormones, ready to respond on command to the trials and tribulations faced by a living organism in an environment that can turn hostile at any moment. So, you've just gotten an unexpected huge tax refund, which you've used to buy a ticket for you and your computer-matched ideal mate to a small island paradise with full-service everything, and are sitting together in the warm sun on a white-sand beach sipping the best drink you both have ever tasted. Life is more than good; it's fricken amazing. Every muscle in your body is relaxed and every internal organ hums with biological balance and bliss. And your natural pacemaker gets the message and your pulse is slow and regular. And being as young and healthy and in love as you are, with potential for procreation and a union of good genes, MN watches with nearly as much ecstasy as you. But then, comes the tsunami, and life suddenly goes from nirvana to shit. And when your eyes see that wave the size of the Hoover Dam approaching and it registers in your brain, your adrenal glands squeeze out a few gallons of hormones, and your pacemaker fires as fast as a humming bird's wings flutter, and you've experienced the miracle of your sinoatrial node's ability to adjust, even if just for a moment.

Alright, our natural pacemaker fires and the top two chambers of our heart (the right atrium transfers its impulse quickly to the left atrium) have received the electrical message and dutifully respond by contracting. The result is blood is pumped, nearly simultaneously, into the two bottom chambers of our heart (the right and left ventricles).

Now what? Well, when the electrical impulse that originated from our natural pacemaker finished its job by causing the contraction of our atria, that impulse is channeled into another very specialized piece of heart tissue that acts as a sentinel of sorts by delaying the electrical impulse before it permits it to enter our two lower heart chambers (the right and left ventricles). This unique "guard" is called the ***atrioventicular node.*** After our atrioventricular node "decides" to permit the impulse to travel on past its checkpoint, the impulse reaches a thick biological "wire" of sorts at the top of our ventricles called the ***bundle of His*** (named after a Swiss cardiologist/anatomist who first discovered it). This thick bundle then divides into two additional thinner, but longer bundles that serve as distribution electrical conduits to the right and left ventricles. The bundle to the right ventricle (thinner) is not surprisingly called the **right bundle branch**, and the bundle to the left ventricle (a lot "beefier" than the right) is called the **left bundle branch**, which has two separate divisions of its own. Now that we're down in the ventricles and the major electrical distance has been covered, there's less need for ultra-fast packaged "wires" and so the additional distribution of the electrical impulse to the remaining part of the ventricles is accomplished by cells that still encourage the rapid distribution of electrical impulses, but are less bundled and are called **Purkinje fibers**.

So now we've got a pretty good idea of the basic structure of the heart and how its valves and conducting system function under normal circumstances. MN should be proud of what she's accomplished, using at least some of the building blocks in the construction of her beloved viruses, algae and bacteria. But her appreciation of our admiration for what she's done is short-lived as she refocuses on some of those who are providing the compliment: abusers of her natural order, whose mutations broke the rules and replaced the sure-footed sleek creatures of her world with the gastronomically obsessed, and the users of mechanical slaves that mock her. So what does she do? She conjures up her revenge, in a partnership with dusty DNA, and introduces the aging human to **atrial fibrillation**.

Remember our natural pacemaker, that precise servant of our biological needs? Well, she (MN) has recognized that she has the option to remove it (physiologically) from the stability equation and substitute total chaos in its place.

What exactly has she done? She's afflicted, generally older people (nearly 3 million current sufferers), with totally random and disorganized impulses from their **atria** (top chambers of their hearts), so that if you could hold those chambers in your hand you would see and feel a sack of writhing worms moving in total disorder. She could have finished the job of removing those individuals from the living if only she hadn't previously installed the ***atrioventricular node*** (remember that "guard" or sentinel that sits between the two upper chambers of the heart and the two lower chambers, processing impulses before letting them pass through?). Well, when this node is bombarded with an infinite number of electrical impulses it says "not so fast", literally. The result of the atrioventricular node's "assessment" is the transmission of a constantly changing, irregularly irregular, generally high number of impulses down to the ventricles, but at a rate (while physiologically, inappropriately fast and often causing symptoms) ***not*** so fast that it deprives the ventricles' ability to send an adequate amount of blood to our lungs and body. If the atrioventricular node did not exist and the infinite number of atrial impulses reached the lower chambers of our hearts, the result would be ***ventricular fibrillation***, which, if not corrected medically or by use of a defibrillator within a few minutes at most, is usually fatal. ***Fibrillating lower chambers can't propel blood*** into the lungs or out to the rest of our organs and tissues.

So, where do we go from here if we're one of those millions of patients with atrial fibrillation, now embraced by many people [whose familiarity with the concept has been nurtured by TV commercials for new blood thinners (see below)] as simply "AF?"

First, if blood in the top chambers of our hearts is supposed to be pushed out into the lower chambers with each heartbeat and it suddenly finds itself swirling around in place, that can't be good. And that's correct. Depending on a number of individual circumstances discussed below, there is a variable but significant risk that the swirling blood may form a ***clot*** along the wall of either top chamber (most likely in an out-pocketing in the left atrium called the ***left atrial appendage***). Once this blood clot forms, it has a tendency to grow and form a tail (like a gelatinous form of an icicle). The tail of the clot may eventually grow long enough to cross the ***mitral valve*** into the ***left ventricle*** where it whips about with each heartbeat. We don't need Murphy's Law to guess what is likely over time. Part, or all, of the tail of the clot breaks off and follows the simple principle that if you toss a stick into the center of a river it's carried with the current; the clot passively does the same thing and usually winds up in the *internal carotid artery* on the way to the *brain* causing a subsequent *stroke*.

Now what? For patients with atrial fibrillation (not occurring as the result of a bad heart valve; this restriction is more to do with the lack of supporting clinical studies than a concrete contraindication), there are ways for the physician to predict the chances of the broken-clot-stroke scenario based on previous observational studies and individual characteristics of the patient in question.

One method (seemingly refined every Tuesday) often used is abbreviated as a ***CHADS2 score***. This looks at certain coexisting and previous conditions and assigns a risk number [CHAD = existing Congestive heart failure, High blood pressure, Age, greater than or equal to 75, Diabetes, and prior Stroke or transient ischemic episode (***TIA***), or blood clot that has broken off from its base in a previous episode, but left no lasting deficit]. For each disease entity that applies to the individual patient, a score of one point is assigned, except for a previous stroke or blood clot, which receives two points. The total number of points is then used to estimate the annual risk of a stroke. For example, a score of 0 in a patient in AF still predicts an annual risk of 1.9%. A score of 6 calculates the risk of stroke at 18.2% in one year. These numbers are guidelines that permit a candid discussion between patient and physician regarding the next step, if any.

Before discussing blood-thinning options that one might choose in the hope of minimizing one's risk for strokes in AF patients with high CHADS2 scores, let me condense an extraordinary complex series of biochemical reactions operational in humans (and frequently responsible for many a medical student falling asleep as if drugged, when the lights turn off in a lecture hall and the projected image appears) by simply suggesting that you imagine a roadmap of the Los Angeles freeway system (subsequently referred to as the "***Freeway Map***").

Assuming you've done that, just accept that every intersection represents a greatly simplified, but distinct and coordinated biochemical reaction that mystically results in a blood clot when the driver has covered every inch on the map. I can present you with an ethereal document that states you know all you have to for this book, accompanied by my suggestion that you don't apply for a fellowship in hematology based on this accomplishment.

Okay, you have ***AF*** and MN is on your ass, trying to punish you for being older than Alice in Wonderland. What do you do? The first step is to have a conversation with your physician with special attention to the risks versus benefit ratio of blood thinning (the term "blood thinner" is technically inaccurate and the word ***anticoagulant*** is preferred). Look, there's always some degree of risk with anything we do. This is true when we eat out in a restaurant, and certainly true when we mess with our biochemistry by introducing a chemical into our system, even if it's FDA approved.

For more than half a century, the medical community only had ***warfarin* (*Coumadin*)** available as an anticoagulant of proven potency to be of value in preventing blood clots from forming or breaking off in patients with "Freeway Map" that ends up in "Clotsville, California." Often referred to as "rat poison" by patients (it was initially introduced for that purpose), it has worked with reasonable efficacy and acceptable bleeding complications.

For years, doctors and patients complained about the need for frequent blood testing (when prescribed warfarin) and the interference with its efficacy when foods containing significant amounts of Vitamin K are consumed. There are prominent genetic factors at play with patients taking this medication. This is not at all surprising when you consider the ***enzymatic steps*** on the "Freeway Map". Some patients require low doses of warfarin (1 mg per day) for stability. The goal is to reach a "thinness" usually expressed as an *International Normalize Ratio* or *INR* in a range of at least 2.0, which simply means that the blood specimen takes twice as long as normal to form a blood clot and that the test for determining the value is universally comparable no matter which lab was used. Other patients require daily doses as high as 12 mg or more to obtain the same effect. Some patients are quite stable, requiring relatively infrequent blood testing; others require frequent testing.

After 50 years with no choice other than warfarin, suddenly our medicine cups runneth over with four new agents and probably more on the way. Whether this bumper crop of agents was just lucky timing, or planned, the new options are welcomed with the growing epidemic of AF as our population ages.

Three of the four new anticoagulants currently approved by the FDA interfere with the journey of a developing clot as it gathers momentum on our "Freeway Map" by "obstructing" its path at a point called *Factor X (ten)*. These agents are: *Xarelto, Eliquis* and *Savaysa*. The fourth agent is *Pradaxa*, which interferes with the final step in coagulation by delaying arrival at "Clotsville," more scientifically referred to as "destination," *thrombin.*

I'm not going to compare the four new additions here except to say that they all work, are usually well tolerated, are somewhat more effective in preventing strokes than warfarin and generally have less potential for causing serious or life threatening bleeding into the brain. For patients well established and stable on warfarin, I see no reason to mess with success.

As you might imagine the competition amongst these new anticoagulant entries is fierce. One undeniable positive result of this combat is that marketing on TV and elsewhere has brought AF into focus for many who were not aware of the ballooning problem, and may now seek medical advice for their skipping or racing heart, which they had previously attributed to too much coffee or listening to the world news.

I cannot neglect another marketing issue of sorts that I feel is generally counter-productive for patients with, or suspicious that they may have, AF. The introduction of these new drugs, and the potential profits they may generate, is like pouring all the blood specimens from a busy lab into an ocean overcrowded with sharks. TV watchers are inundated with law firms advertising their "you-pay-nothing-unless-we-collect" services for those who have suffered significant bleeding complications, or for those whose loved ones experienced a fatal hemorrhage on some of these drugs.

A few quick points: all medications carry some risk; a physician should always discuss the risk/benefit ratio with a patient before starting any new drug, especially an anticoagulant; FDA approval of these anticoagulants for AF involved a careful review of clinical data that compared these new agents to **warfarin** (**Coumadin**) with the conclusion that they were often *more* efficacious in preventing detrimental endpoints, and *less* likely to cause brain hemorrhages; if lawsuits reach the courts, the vast majority are lost by the plaintiff and their attorneys simply because the record will usually reveal that the potential bleeding complications were discussed with the patient, not to mention that the statistical risk of a disabling stroke **without** the anticoagulant in a vulnerable AF patient is far **more likely** to occur than a bleed **on** the medication; understand that an unfortunate adverse reaction is very different from malpractice or negligence; the legal team for the plaintiff hopes that the insurance companies representing the physician or drug company will settle out of court to avoid the time and expense (do this and you might as well dump the whole blood bank into the shark-infested waters); and finally – if you just had neck surgery, are seven months pregnant, have uncontrolled blood pressure and get sea sick when you look at a fish stick, it's probably a smart personal decision **_not_** to ride the world's most outrageous rollercoaster. The point is, ultimately, a reasonably normal, well-informed person must take responsibility for his or her own decisions.

The final question one might ask regarding AF, is how the hell can we prevent it? The short answer is that we're not sure that we can. Medications have mixed, and often temporary, benefits. Realistically these things in our chests (our hearts) have been beating before we had a chest. Our increased longevity has put a burden on all our organs; maybe the first to function should be the first to malfunction? You see, *it's the same old battle I refer to in almost every section: we evolved in a way that placed intelligence above all other survival advantages, and while this has worked well in the short run (in evolutionary terms), there is the risk that everything else in our DNA has never caught up*. Ironically, many electrophysiologists (specialists dealing with the electrochemical functions of our hearts) suggest that our best chance for success may be along the same lines as the origin of our "problem." And maybe the fact that a minimally invasive, closed-chest procedure called **catheter ablation**, which may "cure" AF, and is getting easier and more successful, hints that our intelligence has the potential to find means that will override the lingering disadvantage imbedded in our DNA. But even this procedure, to date, is not always successful, either initially or long term.

Recent work out of Australia followed more than 800 obese men, *all with AF*, for an average of four years. The essential purpose of the study was to assess the effect of various degrees of *weight loss* on the incidence of AF under a variety of therapeutic interventions, including medications, and catheter ablation. Simplifying the results, it appeared that those obese men who lost the most weight (greater than or equal to 10% from baseline) were significantly more likely to remain free of AF (with or without medications and with or without catheter ablation). The results suggest that weight loss alone provides a certain protection against AF; a benefit that persists over and above what one might expect from more standard interventions. (See section: "WHY CAN'T I LOSE WEIGHT? *Obesity and leptin–the human screw-up"*).

Is there a more profound lesson in discussing weight loss again in this section on AF? You bet. ***Here we are in defiance of the natural world with an obesity epidemic and common illnesses unique to our species and in possession of a ton of DNA whose function eludes us. For me, it seems more than likely that the reality of our species' embracing of unnatural selection tempts the secrets still embedded in our genome to run rampant when we scorn the sacred biological balance that struggled to perfection over millions of years***

HAS MY BODY TURNED
AGAINST ME?

Inflammation–overdosing a good thing

L et's go back in time. Let's visit the earliest of our species when, like a toddler today, he or she was having a heck of a time adjusting to the standing position. So, bare-assed or clothed (who knows?), he, or she, on their way to a nearby stream for a drink of water, catches a toe on a tree root and goes down, landing on a knee or elbow in a patch of gravel. Obviously upset, our ancient predecessor rubs the gravel free from his or her bleeding wound, gets that drink, rinses off the blood, and heads back to home base.

Now, let's miniaturize, go microscopic and inside our ancient ancestor. As the skin on an elbow or knee is damaged, a number of cell types (in a sense sitting around and waiting for trouble) get the message through direct damage (skin penetrated, vessels roughed up) and recognize that "bad stuff" on the gravel possess chemistry foreign to what belongs inside our ancient human. These cells (one type of which are called *macrophages*) have receptors on their surfaces that accept the message that something is wrong and respond by releasing substances that initiate a ***protective*** response called ***inflammation***. That's right, when your cat is unhappy that you stopped massaging its neck and bites your hand, the pain, redness, heat and swelling are "good" things MN has provided so that, assuming you're a healthy stud or a ripe-and-ready female, the bite (or a little gravel) won't necessarily infect you, spread into your blood, and eventually kill you, removing perfectly good genes from her pool.

What's happened is that these biochemical reactions to injury have caused tiny blood vessels (***capillaries***) to dilate (thus the redness and warmth) and bring more blood to the damaged site, and in doing so, deploy more infection fighting and healing cells to the battlefront. Also, the ***cell membranes*** (the envelopes that contain the cell's contents) of these capillaries are made more permeable, allowing for the liquid portion of blood (***plasma***) to escape into the damaged area (causing swelling) and bring additional "good" stuff to the site to fight infection and promote healing. Furthermore, within this stew of chemical responders, there are agents that stimulate ***pain receptors***. That's not primarily punishment for stupidity (like a nationally ranked swimmer who, after registering at a hotel a day before competing in the men's 50 freestyle, decides to enter a no-holds-barred kick boxing tournament that evening). No, recognition of pain is a learning experience, which is protective, teaching future avoidance.

So, here we are in modern times and this useful, powerful gift from MN is no longer a done-deal for survival advantage. For example, the inflammatory process is now a known component contributing to the hardening of our arteries (***atherosclerosis***).

Something foreboding seems to have entered our gene pool that can corrupt and harness our inflammatory response as the ultimate example of mistaken identity. ***When our inflammatory responses can no longer differentiate between the crud on a piece of gravel and the protein that is "us," there's a big-time problem***. This so-called ***autoimmunity*** is responsible for a growing number of human diseases involving nearly every organ in our bodies. A few examples are **rheumatoid arthritis**, **lupus erythematosus**, **Type I diabetes** and **Crohn's Disease**.

So what's gone wrong here? How and why has this happened? Here's a clue. You know how a **muscle** gets sore after a vigorous workout? It turns out that such discomfort is, in fact, the result of an **inflammatory process**–the result of microscopic damage. In the repair phase, muscles themselves respond to contraction by apparently synthesizing a number of substances some of which are called **myokines**, which are **peptides** (miniature **proteins** made up of **amino acids** and not usually folded). These **myokines** have effects in the body similar to hormones. Guess what? If that's the case, then skeletal muscle has been graduated to the status of an **endocrine organ** like your **thyroid** and **adrenal glands**! And, there is evidence that one of the effects of these myokines is **anti-inflammatory**!

This opens the possibility that someone in good physical condition (a long-term exerciser, testing muscles in ways elusive to couch sitters) may, through the effects of myokines, protect his or herself from chronic inflammation and the consequences that seem to have afflicted modern humans. It's even possible that regular exercise might play a protective role against autoimmune disease by suppressing or modulating bad genes, and/or "turning on" or modulating good genes.

But there's more. There are a number of ways to measure, or at least estimate, the inflammatory "status" of an individual. **C-reactive protein** (or **CRP)** is a substance made in the liver in response to a chemical alarm sent from cells (remember **macrophages**?) that have been recruited into a "mess" that needed cleaning up as part of the inflammatory response to injury. CRP attaches to the surface of dead cells at the inflamed site as an early step in disposing of the cell debris. So, then blood levels of CRP correlate with what's going on in the body, relative to inflammation, even if not as obvious as those teeth marks left by your puppy.

Guess what? In *obese* patients, there's strong evidence that they are often in a *chronic low-level state of inflammation*. Their CRP values are often high. And there's even evidence that fat cells (*adipocytes*), which are larger in the obese, may lose integrity, triggering an *autoimmune* response not much different than if the offending agent was a piece of gravel.

So, here's the punch line. *Exercising and maintaining a healthy weight is crucial. Inflammation is supposed to be a good thing.* It *was* only a good thing. And while I can't prove it, I'll bet that our early human (or any of his or her relatives, then or in generations that followed) as described at the beginning of this section didn't have a snowball's chance in hell of suffering from hardening of the arteries, diabetes, lupus or rheumatoid arthritis, or any other autoimmune disease. Once again, like no other mutation, the dawn of our superior brainpower extended our lives by unnatural leaps and bounds, the majority of our DNA left in the dust of biological antiquity. And, in that process, we made life as easy as possible, shunning the "work" of regular physical activity and created a whole new set of diseases unknown to our prehistoric ancestors, corrupting inflammation into a potential evil.

There's that "you-get-what-you-pay-for" smirk on MN's metaphoric face.

WHY CAN'T I BREATHE AT NIGHT?

The shape you're in and sleep apnea

Recent discoveries of early human skulls indicate that a number of human species coexisted in our early history, and that we, *Homo sapiens*, are the lone survivors. Thank you MN. What this says is that we obviously had a survival advantage over the others. My guess is that it was intellectual: hunting and gathering with greater success than the losers. Another possibility is adverse mutation, possibly with a dominant pattern of inheritance, which spread the negative trait more quickly from generation to generation, the disadvantage of the physical or biochemical result (whatever it might have been) eventually resulting in the more-vulnerable species' inability to compete and the consequent extinction of its line. Whatever the causes of their failure to thrive, we stand on the top step of the evolutionary podium. And, we did well for the longest of time, our gains in the hunting-and-gathering enterprise ever expanding as fast as our exploding brain capacity. But, living only to forty or fifty seemed unreasonable in the context of our growing dominance over nature. Dysentery, tuberculosis, death during childbirth, are all conquerable foes when the secret weapon is IQ.

Now, here we are, hydrogen bombs in silos, generally well vaccinated, and the masters of our environment, hunting replaced by supermarkets and fast food, and gathering replaced by the Internet and Federal Express. And, in our triumph, too many of us have abandoned the "work" of exercise and the "work" of accepting satiety. And, so many of us, particularly the former hunters, now big and not always tall, have packed on the pounds. Life is too complicated, or unfair, the competition too crafty to "waste" valuable time walking with no purpose other than to use one's muscles and turn on genes that one can't see anyway. And after a hard day of worry (that does not include the risk of starvation), the exhausted corporate (or jobless) warrior retires for yet another lousy night of interrupted sleep.

He lays his head (with its elongated and swollen, soft palate and tongue) on his pillow and, as he drifts into sleep, rolls onto his back and obstructs the passage that connects his nasal cavity to the back of his throat (**nasopharynx**). He obliterates the space where his mouth connects to his airway (**oropharynx**) and, with no open connection between the air in his room and his lungs, stops breathing. **Sleep apnea** has arrived.

And, while no oxygen enters his blood and no carbon dioxide leaves, nasty biochemical changes tax his system (even more than the IRS) and *inch him ever so closer to the consequences, which may include coronary artery disease, heart attack, atrial fibrillation, stroke and diabetes to name a few.*

After seconds to several minutes, his advanced brain can no longer tolerate the bad-news chemistry of his blood and wakes him with a snort that may resemble something his hunting ancestors might have heard when they speared dinner.

Awake now, he's not certain what happened. And, if there is no partner at his beefy side, there is no witness to the event. And so, the next day of persistent repose is accompanied by a mysterious fatigue, which he may mistakenly assume is hypoglycemia and "fixes" it with a Big Mac.

___The lesson here is primarily to recognize the absolute necessity of regular exercise and the need for a valiant attempt at keeping body weight down. Obesity predisposes to sleep apnea___, which can be best diagnosed in special sleep labs, and often successfully treated with the nighttime use of an apparatus called **_Continuous Positive Airway Pressure_**, or **_CPAP._** But, when and if you use CPAP, be certain it has an alarm for a disconnect because MN can be an impatient bitch.

CAN I IMPROVE
MY AGING KNEE JOINTS?

Over the counter and over the top for bad knees

Remember that scene in "Jaws" when the Great White Shark attacks Hooper in the shark cage? Some of that footage was of a real shark, not the notorious mechanical version with its legendary problems. If you watch that scene, you'll notice the violent contortions of the real shark as it gets caught in the cables holding the cage. The shark bends and twists with great force, battering the cage before it finally escapes.

You see, a shark is classified as a ***chondrichthion***, which means its spine is made of ***cartilage*** and connective tissue unlike the boney spine (***vertebral column***) of many other fish (called ***teleosts***). Cartilage is a unique tissue that possesses a number of unusual physical and biochemical properties: to begin with it's flexible and is lighter than bone, advantages for a predatory shark (and no disadvantage to a non-predatory shark) that often must locate, pursue, attack and grab its prey.

I can see MN back before the dawn of man, recognizing that this stuff (cartilage) might have an advantage for a line of creatures she was conditioning for their ascension onto the land and eventual two-legged ambulation. One potential architectural problem for this proposed variant was that this prototypic human must have a pair of lungs that must inflate to fill with air, and must be protected by ribs, a breast bone (***sternum***) and a spine all made of bone (none of these structures exist in sharks), that expands about as easily as a rock. So, MN cleverly alters the blueprint and places *flexible* cartilages at the ends of each rib where they join the sternum. Problem solved with the blessing of the Great Planning Commissioner in the sky. And, while MN preens over one solution, she also realizes that another characteristic of cartilage, its ***resistance to compression***, might make a hell of a good cushion between a *femur* (long leg bone of the thigh) and a ***tibia*** (the thicker lower leg bone – the shin) along with the narrower ***fibula***, which together constitute the lower leg. And so, the stage was set for at least one act in the evolution of the upright human species, not to mention birth of the potential for ***osteoarthritis*** and a lucrative medical specialty called orthopedics.

There are several types of cartilage, but we're going to focus on one type called ***hyaline cartilage***, which is present in many human structures [for example, our noses, rings supporting our windpipes (***tracheae***) and our voice boxes (***larynges***)], and address its structure and function in our ***knees*** in order to try and answer the question: "Is all that money I'm spending on over-the-counter supplements such as ***glucosamine, chondroitin sulfate*** and ***hyaluronic acid*** for my bad knees worth a rat's ass?"

Let's get a bit scientific here (I promise it's necessary to answer the question) and take a microscopic look at the stuff MN decided was the best solution to the wear and tear a terrestrial environment would impose on the knees of upright creatures walking and running in an effort to stay alive.

Best way to look at this is to think of your knee cartilage as a "biological pie." We'll start at the top, where the outer crust sits, and work our way down to the bottom.

First point: there are actually two distinct "pies" of cartilage in "*C*" shapes that sit (and cushion) the junction of the thigh bone (*femur*) as it sits on top of the shin bone (*tibia*). Each of these "C" shaped "pies" of cartilage is called a *meniscus*.

Second point: the very top of our pie, its "crust," is smooth and is the surface that comes in contact with the bone on top of it, the femur (this surface is called the *articular surface*). In our case then, the upper crust of our pie (sitting on top of the shin bone or tibia) makes contact with the lower end of our thighbone or femur.

Now that you're positionally oriented, forget about everything and just focus on the formation of our "pie filling"–actual knee cartilage.

Stem cells (called that because they have the ability to change into different kinds of cells depending on their biochemical environment) migrate to just below the top crust of our knee cartilage and transform into cells that make the "filling" called *chondroblasts*. These "filling-maker" cells do their thing, and as they make filling (more on the recipe for the filling later), they trap themselves in their own product and undergo a transformation into more mature, but less active, "filling makers" called *chondrocytes* (trust me, this stuff is all necessary and really not all that difficult). Okay, these trapped "filling-making" cells can only divide a few times, forming small isolated groups surrounded by fluid-filled *spaces* that are strictly liquid and devoid of the filling. These isolated, trapped islands of a few cells are called *lacunae*. These fluid–filled spaces play a role in facilitating biochemical communication (how much and what quality of filling to make, depending on the body's signals).

Alright, now to the other important ingredients in the "filling," and since we're all experts on the cell types in hyaline cartilage, no more babying: from now on the "filling" in our "pie" will be the *matrix* of our *knee cartilage*.

First of all, the matrix has <u>no</u> nerves and <u>no</u> blood vessels. This means that knee pain is the result of damage in structures other than the cartilage itself. This explains why long-term isolated cartilage damage can go unnoticed. The lack of decent blood supply is a primary reason why damaged cartilage is damn difficult to repair. The matrix itself is very flexible, compressible (with rapid return to baseline configuration), elastic and shock absorbing. So, what is it about the matrix that gives it these advantageous qualities? We need to go biochemical for the answer.

A special group of proteins, called *collagens*, is produced by our *chondrocytes* before and after their entrapment (remember, these trapped islands of cells and the fluid contained within them are called lacunae). These proteins are produced as fibrils. For now, think of these molecular structures as *thin flexible rods of amino acids* with properties that make them just "dying" to hook up and tangle with the right passerby.

Next, on to *glucosamine*. Sound familiar? This is a sugar-like substance that not only appears on the label of the bottle you just purchased to supposedly help your arthritis pain, but is found extensively in the shells of shellfish and the protective coverings of insects. All that you need know about it until the next paragraph is that it is a chemical *precursor* (a substance that will be biochemically transformed before it reaches its intended structure and function).

Chondroitin sulfate and *hyaluronic acid* are both amino acids hooked up to sugars (they both share the nasty name of *glycosaminoglycan* or *GAG* – no, it's not supposed to be funny, that's really its name). The glucosamine, just mentioned in the previous paragraph will be altered and eventually join chondroitin sulfate and hyaluronic acid as a glycosaminoglycan (remember, it's just amino acids hooked up to sugars).

Okay, so we've got most of the ingredients in this matrix (our pie filling) with these nests of cells (***chondrocytes***) isolated in small groups in that hunk of cartilage that prevents bone-on-bone trauma when we jog (or finally decide to walk into a fast-food restaurant when the line of cars at the drive-through is too long).

Now what? Well, MN "mixes" the biological stew and things happen: the ***hyaluronic acid forms a backbone*** of bottle-brush-like mega molecules with linkages to "arms" of protein from which many molecules of chondroitin sulfate hook up (like pine-needle branches), which form aggregates (called ***aggrecans***–creative, huh?) that make the whole conglomerate look like a ***molecular junk yard full of those ancient TV antennae***. But there's more: all that "hungry" collagen "sitting around" finds its destiny and ties up the junk-yard of antennae with its own extensive fibrils. And, from all that "apparent" chaos, one of the chemical characteristics of our "fibril-bound," over-the-counter supplements pulls in a ton of water, flooding our "junk yard" such that knee cartilage is about 70% water, a component essential for the safe movement of two intimately contacting bones!

MN looks over her work and is pleased. The end result of all I have very simply (believe it or not) outlined is a shock-absorbing knee cartilage that does everything she wanted it to do. Now, get out there young stud with all those good genes and run down a mate of equal-quality DNA, and be fruitful and multiply. But, when MN sees the grimacing post-prime hobblers sway with a gait that screams knee dysfunction and/or pain, she loses her smile and wonders if she might find a way to place twice as many concrete barriers in the parking lots of malls to facilitate a devastating hip facture!

Let's get practical. It's estimated that about 10% of the entire US population over 18 takes a glucosamine supplement for one reason or another. Worldwide, billions are spent yearly on glucosamine. It is true that radio-isotope-tagged glucosamine supplements do, in fact, wind up in our joints.

There are two theories speculating on how any of the above-mentioned OTC products might work on knees to reduce pain and/or inflammation, improve mobility and/or flexibility, or heal or prevent deterioration of cartilage.

The first theory basically suggests that by *"overloading" the system* with lots of raw materials, you'll push the biochemical process into a more active state. For me, that's like dumping a truckload of straw at the feet of a basket weaver, already working at full capacity, and demanding more finished product.

The second theory is that these OTC products play an *anti-inflammatory role* that either helps mend damaged cartilage, or minimizes its deterioration. If one evokes the counter argument that lots of other anti-inflammatory remedies exist (including OTC non-steroidal anti-inflammatory agents such as *Motrin*, *Advil* and *Aleve*, known as *NSAIDs*), and that the data on the long-term effects of these on the process of osteoarthritis is mixed at best, a legitimate challenge might be that those products failed only because they were not as intimately connected to the biochemistry of knee cartilage. It's a tough point to counter, even though I intuitively doubt its validity.

All this having been said, there are more impressive studies suggesting glucosamine's (and the other OTC's mentioned, fairly or not, by association) *failure* to objectively improve or halt cartilage deterioration in osteoarthritis, than studies to the contrary.

One study, for example, was well controlled and did *not* show any benefit over placebo by MRI scan after six months of therapy with glucosamine. When you examine *the intimate chemical relationship of glucosamine, chondroitin sulfate, and hyaluronic acid in the molecular matrix ("junk yard") that gives hyaline cartilage its unique properties, it intuitively seems reasonable (admittedly not very scientific) to assume that if glucosamine doesn't work, the chances are neither will chondroitin sulfate nor hyaluronic acid.*

There are **surgical procedures** available (usually for athletically induced cartilage damage) that attempt to stimulate new cartilage production by drilling tiny holes in bone.

Stem cell research is always looking for a way to introduce these multi-potential cells with the hope that they will do exactly the right thing when you place them where the trouble is. Still waiting on that.

It's important to realize that when research results are either conflicting or ambiguous, the proposed therapy is most likely not a magic bullet like a successful appendectomy for a bad appendix. So, <u>*my recommendation is that glucosamine, chondroitin, and hyaluronic acid in the usual OTC amounts suggested on the label are unlikely to do any harm (except to your wallet), and nearly as unlikely to do any good*</u>.

The exception might be that someone suffering with **osteoarthritis** of the fingers, who develops often painful, bony swellings in the finger joints (called **Heberden's nodes**), arising from repeated trauma to cartilage and the "corrective" response of "filling in" the defects with excessive bone production might, theoretically, slow the process (not reverse or cure it) by reducing cartilage deterioration with these supplements. Still no final answer on this.

Finally, I would be remiss if I didn't mention one very **unscientific** buzz that tends to haunt my loyalty to the scientific method. Many veterinarians swear that they often see impressive results when they place older, arthritic dogs on one or more of these supplements. Since the dog didn't pay good money for the pills (and is unlikely to fully comprehend how pleasing it would be for its master to enter it in an agility contest when it currently has to be lifted manually into the back of the pickup), it's unlikely to be influenced by the placebo effect. After factoring in the unexplored possibility that the vets I've spoken to may sell the supplements, one can come to one's own conclusions.

The purpose of cartilage, according to MN's rules, was to serve us for probably no more than four our five decades, a reality that our DNA will not overlook. Cartilage does respond positively to appropriate forces applied to it. If cartilage is there to do a specific job, continuous, conservative deployment of that function is more than likely to help sustain it in the best condition biologically possible. Inactivity can only send the message to our DNA that we no longer require the services of this remarkable substance. And also remember that MN probably sees the perpetually motionless the same as she sees the dead.

WHAT'S THE DEAL WITH BARIATRIC SURGERY?

Evolutionary impatience

So here you are, an ancient fish happily eating your usual diet (whatever that might have been), as the current occasionally carries a batch of tempting morsels close enough for one of your senses to pick it up on radar. Then you pursue it, snatch it up in your mouth, swallow it, and digest it for its life-sustaining nutrition. Ahh, life is good. But then, one day, or one thousand years later, alas, the currents brought only unappetizing stuff of a different sort and a new and unexpected challenge arose: better start learning to eat things you may not prefer or die.

Helped along by random mutations that made the task of adjusting to a new diet either more palatable, and/or biologically more beneficial, some individuals made the accommodation. Others though, may have failed and MN, with no intended malice, simply removed their maladjusted asses from the ranks of her more favored children. And over time, for some of these mutated fish, their requirement for protein may have lessened, or their intestines may have developed greater efficiency, or they may have adjusted to constant grazing for food in the sand on the ocean floor or the muck that covers the bottom of lakes, with the result that *they no longer needed stomachs*. In other words, when a distinct stomach was no longer a survival advantage, their DNA was no longer "encouraged" to retain the genes that make stomachs, and consequently "disposed" of them over time.

Most vertebrates however, mammals in particular, do possess a *stomach*. Certain groups–called *ruminants*–such as cows and goats have multi-chambered stomachs to accommodate their particular mode of eating and diet. The stomach is an obvious evolutionary development with *survival advantage* (just as the loss of a stomach was no evolutionary *disadvantage* in my earlier example).

A jaguar may search for weeks without finding prey. When it finally does and makes its kill, it has to really fill up if it hopes to survive. Without a stomach, the cat would feel full after consuming only a small amount; the remaining portion of the kill would be subject to predation by competing carnivores, scavengers or it might just rot and add nitrogen to the earth. In the case of our jaguar, its stomach functions more than just a "storage" organ. It is an important source of digestive enzymes such as *pepsin*, *hydrochloric acid*, and the hormone *gastrin*, all of which are needed to digest, or partially digest, protein, carbohydrates, and fats.

Of course, the process of digestion in cats <u>and</u> humans begins in the *mouth*. Chewing increases the surface area of food, and our saliva adds the enzymes *lipase* and *amylase* for early fat digestion.

After the *stomach* empties, the upper part of the small intestine (called the *duodenum*) produces *hormones and hormone-like substances*, which regulate functional activities in the stomach, gallbladder and pancreas. The *gall bladder* responds to hormones from the *duodenum* by contracting and sending its *bile* (which acts as a detergent to help break up fat) into the duodenum. The *pancreas* also responds to signals from the *duodenum* and adds *enzymes* to the mix, the results include the neutralization of acid from the stomach, further degrading of protein and fat, the breaking up of starch and glycogen, and even the digestion of DNA and RNA present in the food that was consumed.

Okay, that's a scaled-down physiology course in human digestion. What's worth noting is that the system is, a priori, biologically efficient because if it weren't, MN's lieutenant (*natural selection*) wouldn't have let it happen.

So, now let's go back and make a comparison between our original blissful fish with a stomach and its seemingly lifetime free pass to the underwater Cheese Cake Factory. Assume for a moment that the balance of nature in the body of water in which our fish lived got shaken up and the current delivered its food source *continuously* rather than *occasionally* (the Cheese Cake Factory changed its business hours to open all day and all night). Stomach full, our fish's brain would hormonally signal "satiety" and our fish would stop eating. The excess, uneaten food would be available with a number of potential biological consequences: for example, better nourished, stronger healthier parents might make more fertile eggs with a higher percent of hatching; more baby fish might grow faster and fitter and thus avoid predation. Whatever the consequences, a balance would be restored with no detriment to the species involved (including the food source itself, which, for example, might benefit from mutations that might allow it to reproduce more effectively or swim more evasively.) *Balance, balance, balance. It drives the inevitable progression of mutation-based evolution in the natural world.*

Enter humans, with our expanded intelligence, who throw a wrench into the works and infuriate MN. So, here we are, and suddenly the Cheese-Cake-Factory metaphor transforms into reality. Our modified brains don't necessarily respond to *leptin* (see section: "WHY CAN'T I LOSE WEIGHT? *Obesity and Leptin–the human screw-up*"). We create the unnatural state of 24/7 access to food. We subject ourselves to Pavlovian-savy marketing, and we fall victim to the distinctly human, self-deceiving concept that it's only the other guy, or gal, who's vulnerable to statistics as we get fat in record numbers, and get depressed with the thought of the most uncomfortable chore of dealing with hunger by abstention.

So, here we are in this expanding epidemic of obesity and all that MN can do about it is hope that we will explode. But our intelligence comes to the rescue with an idea that previously only evolution could have considered as a very long-term solution through mutation and natural selection. Let's change our guts! Not through the unacceptably long and laborious method employed by nature, but nearly instantly. ***Patience is only a virtue if you have time for it.***

As a horrified MN looks on, surgeons, those master mechanics of human machinery, ***design methods to solve the problem*** of terminal fast food by shielding calories from absorption and sending them (along with supplements of some good stuff that you really do need), mainly unabsorbed, out into the Neverland of city sewers and septic tanks.

These "***solutions***" vary from some substantially re-routed plumbing to temporary barriers to intestinal absorption. The general recommendations for consideration for these procedures include possessing a ***Body Mass Index*** (or ***BMI***) of ***40 or more***. This is calculated as mass in kilograms divided by height in meters squared, or mass in pounds divided by height in inches squared and then multiplied by the number 703.

To give you a more realistic idea as to how big you have to be for candidacy, ***a 40-BMI person would stand 5 feet, 2 inches and weigh 219 pounds***. Some patients, particularly with associated medical problems such as high blood pressure, or diabetes, or high "bad" cholesterol (***LDL***), may be considered for the interventions with BMI's as low as the ***low 30's***.

While there are non-surgical procedures, involving the insertion of devices through a scope into the stomach (a balloon previously removed from the market, but making a comeback in a modified form, is still not approved in the USA), or into the small bowel (called an ***endoluminal sleeve***), I will focus on a single, invasive procedure because, frankly, its radical nature (in a biological sense) must drive MN nuts. This is not because I wish her undeserved consternation for doing her job, but rather a vivid example of how human ingenuity so often, intentionally or not, defies the natural world.

The most frequently performed bariatric surgical intervention is called a ***Roux-n-Y procedure*** and is performed either by opening the belly for direct access to one's organs, whose anatomical relationships will be revised, or, with the assistance of a special scope (***laparoscope***), which is introduced through a series of small holes in the abdominal wall, allowing the surgeon to see your internal anatomy ***indirectly*** on a screen from which he does his stuff. Here's what's done.

First, the top of the ***stomach*** is separated from the body of the stomach. The ***walnut-sized*** upper piece of stomach that is attached to the ***esophagus*** is now the only storage for food as it is eaten. Not room for much. Forget about that burger you could hardly get your mouth around–now, not much than a pickle slice or two will fit.

Okay, now what? Well, those pickle slices have to go somewhere, so the surgeon makes an escape route for them by cutting into the ***small bowel*** and bringing it up to the walnut-size pouch and then hooking the two together in a ***side-to-side union***. Now that very satisfying reduced volume of food can work its way out of its solitary confinement and enter the small bowel.

But, more plumbing is necessary because by bringing up the small bowel for the pickle exit, the bigger, lower part of the stomach (which has been closed off from the reduced, remaining functional stomach (the walnut) still makes its "juices," which must have their own biologically sound exit. Remember, by cutting into the small bowel to bring it up to our new mini-stomach, we've got an open-end piece of bowel into which, if the remaining larger part of the stomach dumped its contents, they would pour into our abdominal cavity, creating as much havoc (tissue damage from enzymes and infection) as if someone ran a saber through one's bowel; this is not an acceptable outcome. *The surgeon avoids this potential catastrophe by joining the open-ended piece of small bowel back into a different portion of the small bowel from which it came. So, try and picture this puzzle: tiny stomach with connection to small bowel; open end of small bowel created by the joining of the bowel to tiny stomach reinserted into another portion of small bowel, which allows larger lower piece of stomach to dump contents it still makes into small bowel avoiding disaster.*

Now test your spatial brain power (not to mention your imagination): visualize the section of the bowel that was brought up to the small stomach pouch. Now focus on a section somewhere below the remaining larger part of the stomach and assume it's bent just a bit into sort of a "U" shape. Now picture the piece of bowel attached to the lower, larger stomach pouch that we hooked up to the small bowel to prevent the stomach contents from dumping into our abdominal cavity. But, specifically join it to the small bowel right at the trough of the "U" shaped bowel we just visualized. Get it? We sort of made a "Y." And, thus the name of the procedure (talk about poetic license!), and a mild headache for my devoted readers. Almost done. One final road-map issue. If you are exceptionally gifted spatially, and can actually picture what the surgeon has done, you will notice that the reduced volume of food in the small pouch that was formed will travel through the small bowel in a fashion that *bypasses* a significant portion of the nutrient absorbing bowel. So you see, *not only does the post-operative patient feel full very quickly with small amounts of food, but that small amount of ingested nutrition is further subjected to decreased absorption resulting in a double whammy of calorie reduction!*

Now when *the Roux-n-Y procedure* is completed, the post-op patient must deal with a significant adjustment period. At first, while still in hospital, only small amounts of liquids are permitted. Well-trained personnel will guide the patient through progressive steps leading to more "normal" food ingestion. But, things will never quite be the same as nature intended. While some reversals of the procedure may be possible, such interventions carry significant risks. This is one reason why the patient's pre-op, psychological status is important in determining candidacy. With such deliberate nutritional compromise, in addition to the goal of weight loss, there is the obvious concern for adequate intake and absorption of key elements essential for health. This is accomplished with supplements, as I alluded to earlier in this section.

Studies have shown major clinical benefits from the Roux-n-Y procedure over relatively long periods of time. *The most impressive improvements in prognosis have been seen in patients with obesity-associated medical problems such as hypertension and diabetes.*

So, this bariatric surgery does work. But don't fool yourself; it works because we've so devastatingly suffered from the consequences of out-dated DNA playing its nasty tricks in our species' aging gene pool (MN might call her once beloved accomplishment, more a cesspool) that one solution may necessitate aggressive, unnatural tactics.

A "greener" solution to the insidious predicament that afflicts our species is to recognize the problem and potential problems early on and devote one's self (or advise one's children or grandchildren) of preventive measures, such as an appropriate regimen of *regular physical exercise (from the time you demonstrate the sucking reflex until the time you can no longer perform the maneuver on command), and a diet rich in lean protein, high fiber, monosaturated fats, whole grains, fruits and vegetables, and low in cotton-candy.* Once again: try to fool MN, rather than shock her.

IS DIZZY DANGEROUS?

The balance of balance

Let's start by creating a fictional early super human who was a physical marvel, but still dumb as mud. This guy, or gal, had the reflexes of a cat and the strength of a dead-lift champion with none of the bulk. He or she moved with grace and speed whether walking or running across sandy or muddy terrain, or climbing or swinging from branch to branch in this artificial, nonsensical environment I've fashioned to make a point. But I've made him or her most remarkable in ways that are both not obvious and applicable to modern *Homo sapiens,* as you will soon see.

These creatures had it all: a stable community with plenty of food and water, and no enemies. That is, until one day when a uniquely mean-spirited, sub-human flesh eating, and starving loner appeared out of nowhere. This "mega mess of meanness" foamed at the mouth when it saw what appeared a smorgasbord of lesser victims waiting like defenseless main courses. So, it attacked. And attacked. And, after a while, it was so exhausted, not to mention hypoglycemic, that it could barely haul its frazzled ass back to where it had come.

Here's what happened when anyone of our good guys or gals (or for that matter any of us in 2015, assuming a physiologically functional anatomy needed for balance) were threatened. They saw the bad guy. Their eyes transmitted the image to their *retina* in which specialized cells sensed the light (the image of the bad guy). In low light cells called *rods* were activated, and in brighter light cells called *cones* were stimulated and provided information perceived as color discrimination. In addition, the retinal image categorized the orientation of objects in the environment (what's in the vicinity of the bad guy and what is vertical and what is horizontal). All this visual info is sent to the brain, including a special part called the *cerebellum.*

At the same time as the bad-guy's image was sensed, our good protagonist cocked his or her head in a moment of surprise. This tiny movement triggered a heck of a response. The *inner ear* (go deeper beyond your ear drum into a hollowed out portion of skull and you'll find this remarkable organ) was able to appreciate this head tilt. This inner ear, in particular what is called the *vestibular mechanism* or *system* is an organ that looks like the child of an octopus and a snail. Picture this: take three arms of an octopus and insert their ends back into the body of the octopus, forming loops. But, orient each of these loops at 90 degrees to each other (this portion of the inner ear is called the *semicircular canals*, and is filled with a liquid called *endolymph*). Now elongate the body of the octopus (this "stretched" central portion is called the *vestibule*) and at its very end curl it up into concentric circles like the shell of a snail (this portion is called the *cochlea*). If you have trouble constructing this image, just Google the damn thing under "inner ear."

Okay, I'll assume you have a reasonable picture of what the inner ear looks like (this really is important and has practical applications as you will see, so take a moment to get it and maybe avoid an unnecessary visit to an emergency room where you might wait long enough to actually evolve).

One final addition to our image of your inner ear: in the elongated or "stretched" portion (the vestibule), there are two specialized areas, which have additional function. They are called the *saccule* and the *utricle*. Both of these have an unusual microscopic structure, which includes a membrane (called an *otolithic membrane*) with *calcium carbonate crystals* embedded in it. Now, file all this anatomy along with what we said earlier about the *rods* and *cones* of the eye's retina and the transmission of the image and orientation of the bad guy's position to the part of our brain we've labeled the *cerebellum.*

Back to our bad guy and our protagonists' initial response to the unexpected threat. Okay, protagonist sees bad guy and the image registers. Good guy, or gal, cocks his or her head in a moment of surprise, then glances left and right, surveying the environment in preparation for escape. Good guy, or gal, then leans just a bit forward onto the balls of his or her feet, creating a slight change in pressure on skin, knees, hips and lower back in preparation for a run to safety. Every one of these slight adjustments in body posture have been sensed by special receptors (called *proprioreceptors*) in skin, joints, and muscle (just like pain or temperature receptors) that record the change and by way of the *spinal cord* sent their messages back to the same place in the brain that received the visual image–the *cerebellum.*

Now to the actual escape. Our good guys flee in every direction, some onto sandy terrain, some into mud, others across rocky surfaces. Many double back and find their feet adjusting to a different surface than the one they first encountered. What seems unusual is that when we clock their speed or analyze their running form in slow motion on various running surfaces, nothing changes. It seems our fictional superhuman good guys, or gals, make instant adjustments to any surface.

Now, even angrier, our mega monster, a capable climber, drives his prey into the trees. But the good guys, or gals, put on an acrobatic show that would make Barnum & Bailey blush with envy. Our protagonists swing from branch to branch, ascend and descend, blindly catch branches as if they were extensions of their own limbs, and perform 360-degree somersaults with precision.

Defeated, dizzy and nauseated from watching the antics of his would-be victims, the Godzilla of sub-humanity retires to vomit in peace and never return.

Alright, what's the point (besides the bedtime story you might tell a precocious five-year-old interested in anthropology)? Here's what's important: humans are the evolutionary recipients of a truly remarkable, and complicated, system that maintains our balance. Think about it. What chance in hell does any creature have for survival if it walks around or runs like it's wasted with booze? So, when you, or just your eyes, move, there is a coordinated response to keep both your perception and physical posture compensated.

Here's a quick **summary** of what happened during our protagonists' escape (and still happens in modern *Homo sapiens)*: eyes see bad guy–retina registers bad guy's position and yours (where you and it stands); image of bad guy sent to cerebellum and other parts of brain; you posture in preparation for escape–proprioreceptors in joints, muscles and skin sense the prelude to escape and send their message up the spinal cord to the cerebellum; you run–your *horizontal acceleration* is sensed by the **utricle** in your inner ear, which sends its message back to your cerebellum, and propriore-ceptors (mainly in your ankles) determine the terrain, and send this message up the spine to various parts of the brain, which sends new instructions back down the spinal cord, adjusting your running style accordingly (practice strengthens and better coor-dinates body position and the compensation needed); you quickly climb a tree–the **saccule** in your inner ear detects the *vertical ac-celeration* and sends the message to your cerebellum; you turn your head **down** to see the position of the predator, then **up** and then **left** and **right**, surveying the branches–the **endolymph** in all three of your **semicircular canals** (the "octopus" arms folded back to form loops) detect all head motions and send the information to your cerebellum; you do a 360-degree somersault and just about everything mentioned in this summary gets the message and sends the information to the parts of your brain necessary for your posture and muscles to adjust so you don't fall on your ass. You must admit this is really quite amazing!

So, when a patient comes into my office and complains of "dizziness" and expects, rightfully, if not naively, a simple answer, you can see why I might fantasize, for just a second, what a dermatology residency would have been like.

Back to reality and the first clinical distinction I must make: Is the patient's complaint accurately "*dizziness*," or does he, or she, really mean "*vertigo?*" For purposes of this section, I will assume that neither symptom is part of a clinical picture suggestive of a transient reduction in blood supply to certain parts of the brain (called *TIA*), which may present with similar complaints.

Dizziness is a feeling of instability while you stand, as if you might fall if you stepped forward. Lots of reasons for true dizziness, but, particularly in older patients, they're often over-medicated with blood pressure-lowering drugs (see section: "IS LOWER BLOOD PRESSURE ALWAYS BETTER? *Going beyond therapeutic?*"). True vertigo, on the other hand, is often related to something amiss in the vestibular system, which we have just outlined risking coma in my readers. *Vertigo is accompanied by the sensation that your environment is in motion when you are not.* Uncontrollable eye movements in various directions (called *nystagmus*) are not infrequently clinically evident.

Okay, MN has given us this extremely complicated, but beautifully coordinated and effective, means to know where our bodies and heads are. This gift is particularly helpful in hostile situations (sudden gust of wind while we walk on a frozen sidewalk or the return of a modern version of our angry beast) where that information is essential for both our comfort and/or our survival.

But, remember, MN is proud of her work only in the context that it benefits the young and reproductively capable. It's clear that MN realizes that vertigo is not a real plus if a youthful, romantic male with good genes gets down on his knees to propose to an equally genetically desirable female, then stands, blissful with her acceptance, then suddenly, overcome by a spinning world, vomits, as she recants her acceptance. One must wonder if MN, relying on the innocent but brutal rules in her playbook, designed the human balancing mechanism with purposeful profundity. Hey look, seems pretty obvious that a good way to eliminate the food consumption by a guy with dried up testes and a woman with pin-point ovaries (if any) is to implant a multi-faceted, but delicate, mechanism for survival, suited for the young and biochemically sound, with a built-in expiration date (say forty or fifty years max) so that aged human specimens, resistant to annihilation through their damned-smart grasp of chemistry, will stagger, fall, break a hip or at least aspirate and die of pneumonia.

So, what do we, the post-forty or fifty group, do? I would suggest that there's an unintended "weakness" in MN's predisposition to thoroughness. We should recognize that there is an opportunity in the multiple inputs that help control our balance. ***We can train one system to help override any deficiency in another***.

In the past when I jogged on country roads, I would occasionally turn my head quickly in response to the sudden and unexpected sound of a barking dog, uncertain whether the pooch was safely behind a fence or a stray with rabies. My sudden head movement, especially after miles run in hot weather, occasionally provoked a true vertigo. At first, I sat down on the roadside and let it pass, usually in a few minutes. But, then I decided to try something more proactive. When it happened subsequently, I forced myself to focus on a stable distant object, such as a stop sign, and, no matter how I swayed on the road, no matter how many people thought I was drunk, I continued onward. After a number of trials, I could stop the vertigo in seconds, not minutes. You see, what I did was ***train*** the important visual component in the process of balance to play a greater role.

Another "trick" I've learned through experience utilizes an ***elliptical trainer.*** What I do is ***close my eyes*** (the elliptical hand grips and stable footing allows this) and then, while still exercising, I quickly turn my head to the left, then to the right and then forward. This is repeated with variation (might turn left, then forward, then repeat left, for example). What I'm doing here is eliminating the important visual input and by doing so I'm training my ***proprioreceptors*** to play a greater role.

You need not jog or have any equipment to accomplish the same results by practicing your balance. You can stand on one leg, walk a narrow beam (at ground level, please), use an inflated balance ball for core-muscle propriorceptive training, or enroll in yoga or tai chi classes. <u>Engage in any activity that forces your body to adjust to changes in position with a corresponding correction to maintain stability</u>. Remember, MN doesn't frown on the concept of training because it blinds and deafens her to the biological reality of aging.

SUMMARY AND CONCLUSIONS

W hat I have tried to do in this book, after decades of private medical practice in a closely knit community, is more than provide the reader with practical advice on a variety of subjects commonly requested by my patients, many of whom have become friends. My purpose is to address *the reality that our egos (an understanding of who and where we are) function in a universe of incomprehensible size and complexity; and that a similar universe, no less complex, resides in us. So, in a sense, a "normal" person must elect to see his or herself as the master of both worlds, rather than trapped between them.* This is both healthy and intended by Mother Nature.

But, she (or the force that created her) sees us in more finite terms. She bears us no personal animosity. She is a "bitch" only in the sense that she refuses to recognize our individuality, seeing us only as a species, created, or evolved, or both, for the purpose of maintaining a balanced world. For her, a member who violates this balance should be dead meat. And for this balance to work, for the planet to survive, functioning in the reality of ticking time, there must be accommodation for change. Spontaneous mutation is just that – impromptu. These alterations in the biological status quo are inevitable, but expected to self-regulate by natural selection – and the beat goes on, with no expected change in tempo.

Over time, big alterations in size and shape and biochemistry are expected, welcomed by a doting MN. But then something suddenly (in evolutionary terms) catches MN's eye and raises suspicion. The genetic product isn't particularly fast or strong, but it survives by cunning rather than physical prowess. Still, not alarmed, MN watches and waits for the balance, as human disease doesn't disappoint for long. She's content to watch the birth of an effective immune system so long as enough less-adaptive victims still die from infection. She's equally content to watch some of the females of the species die in childbirth, the survivors of both circumstances (immune competency and surviving mom) part of the plan of natural selection.

But, then something else happens. Over millions of years, an instant in MN's book, mutated genes that should shove the owners towards elimination from the gene pool, are overridden by cleverness. And, as these dormant "cancers" accumulate in the species' genome, MN looks on in horror. But, she has one ally that will not desert her: the built-in time clock that exists in every genome, whether it's a newborn human, an 80-year-old tortoise, or a 1000 year old redwood.

Living forever without changing is contrary to the essence of life; it's the "price" paid for the concession nature grants for inhabiting the planet with more feeling than a piece of granite. While MN watches with disdain as our species lives on with heart disease, emphysema, diabetes, hypertension, obesity and a variety of other diseases–some so alien to her plan that some of her creatures may even fail to recognize their own protein as self–she laments. Ignorant of political turmoil (not her thing), MN waits and hopes that somehow the good old days of meaningful natural selection will return.

Remember though, <u>*Mother Nature is a metaphor for all that is in our DNA and its timed deterioration intended to favor the young and reproductive*</u>. *Mother Nature's fickleness is our chance to turn on good genes (or modulating substances with benefit), and turn off bad genes (or modulating substances with ill effects) with targeted behavior.* In a sense, I have played the role of MN's psychiatrist, probing her history (evolution) and, calling on my medical experience as both a clinician and a journal junkie, trying to speculate how our species might fool her, permitting both a longer and a more superior quality life than she ever intended.

<u>*My assumption throughout this book has been that there's enough plasticity in our DNA to allow us, with adequate science and a little common sense, to still deceive her.*</u> *So long as you keep in step with her double-time march of youth, she may not notice you. But, even with a lifetime of compliance with her drumbeat pace, one hesitation, one relaxed, savoring moment of self-satisfying accomplishment and rest, and she may spot you. And, then there's the real risk that you've shaken her confidence in your value, and she might realize that you are aging, branding you unworthy in an evolutionary sense.*

www.ingramcontent.com/pod-product-compliance
Lightning Source LLC
Chambersburg PA
CBHW031208270326
41931CB00006B/474